S0-BXT-704

MEDICAL TECHNOLOGY, HEALTH CARE AND THE CONSUMER

MEDICAL TECHNOLOGY, HEALTH CARE AND THE CONSUMER

Edited by

Allen D. Spiegel, Ph.D.

Downstate Medical Center
State University of New York
Brooklyn, N.Y.

Donald Rubin
Shelley B. Frost

Consumer Commission on the Accreditation of
Health Services, Inc.
New York

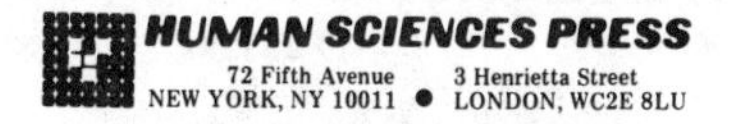

Published by Human Sciences Press, Inc.
72 Fifth Avenue, New York, New York 10011

Printed in the United States of America
123456789 987654321

Library of Congress Cataloging in Publication Data

Main entry under title:

Medical technology, health care and the consumer.

Includes bibliographical references and index.
1. Medical care—United States—Congresses. 2. Medical policy—United States—Citizen participation—Congresses. 3. Medical instruments and apparatus—Evaluation—Congresses. 4. Medical innovations—Evaluation—Congresses. 5. Medical innovations—Economic aspects—United States—Congresses.
I. Spiegel, Allen D. II. Rubin, Donald. III. Frost, Shelley B. IV. Consumer Commission on the Accreditation of Health Services
RA395.A3M44 362.1'0973 LC 79-25559
ISBN 0-87705-498-3

CONTENTS

PREFACE

Health care consumers now serve on governing boards of local, state, and national health planning agencies as required by legislation. In this capacity, consumers are regularly making health policy decisions. Many of these decisions are related directly to the introduction of sophisticated medical technologies into the health care delivery system. Despite the fact that consumers may not be knowledgeable about health care issues and services, they are involved equally with the expert in decision making. In fact, federal health planning legislation calls specifically for consumers who are not involved with the health care industry to be in the majority on the governing boards of health planning agencies. This situation creates a problem in providing adequate, understandable information to those consumers thrust into unaccustomed policy-making roles.

This book is one outcome of a project which attempted to address the issue of medical technology and the consumer. The project was created and sponsored by the Consumer Commission on the Accreditation of Health Services, Inc. and supported primarily by the Science for Citizens program of the

National Science Foundation (Grant No. OSS-7720845). Project objectives included the following:

To provide accurate and reliable information about technological and scientific advances in health care to consumers involved in decisions about those advances and their relation to the health care delivery system.

To inform consumers about the issues related to quality care assessment and to cost/benefit evaluations regarding the increased use of medical technology and the impact of such use on medical and hospital delivery systems.

To stimulate the receptiveness of health care providers to consumer participation by increasing the substantive knowledge of consumers presently involved in the health care decision-making processes.

To develop a manual that could be used by consumer decision makers in evaluating medical technology.

To achieve these objectives, four all-day conferences were scheduled during the latter part of 1978. Each conference format called for a morning session in which speakers made presentations to the audience and responded to questions. Afternoon sessions included workshops at which participants and presenters were able to engage in an exchange of ideas and information. Each conference had a different theme as noted below:

June 17, 1978—Medical Technology and the Health Care Consumer

September 16, 1978—The Impact of Medical Technology on Sickness and Death

October 21, 1978—The Economics of Medical Technology

November 18, 1978—The Future of Medical Technology

Intensive effort was devoted to presenting a balanced point of view about the health care system and its problems relative to consumers. Staff members and the Project Advisory Committee (identified in the lists on pp. 23–29) sought to bring together health economists, public health specialists, private practice health care providers, health lawyers, medical scientists, and third-party payers with consumer advocates and community people involved in health policy-making activities. Information exchange and consciousness raising were important features of the conference series. Both consumers and providers were asked to consider the social, economic, and ethical issues bearing upon the use of medical technology in the health care system and the legislative health planning mandates to develop a rational comprehensive system.

Since the mid-1960s, there was a significant expansion in the concept of community participation in health care policy making. Experts no longer exclusively determine the allocation of health resources; consumers play a vital role in those determinations. However, issues relating to health care decisions have become more and more complex over the years creating difficulties for experts and consumers alike. Today, any scientist or consumer who wishes to make informed decisions faces an intellectual challenge in understanding the implications of adopting complex medical technologies.

Response to the conference series was enthusiastic, testifying to the need and desire to exchange views and to clarify the social and scientific problems raised by medical technology. Mailings and conference announcements drew hundreds of registrants from the ranks of consumers as well as providers. Consumers came from community health centers, voluntary health organizations, trade unions, consumer health groups, hospital advisory boards, and from the local and state health planning agencies of New York and surrounding areas. Health care providers, including private physicians, scientists, health planners, hospital administrators, economists, and third-party insurance administrators also attended in large numbers. Speakers and panel members were nationally recognized in their fields and locally prominent. Many organizations were helpful in developing the program content and in making conference arrangements. Verbal and written evaluations overwhelmingly endorsed the series and expressed the hope that similar conferences would take place in the future.

Addresses presented at the morning sessions of the four conferences are reproduced in this book. In addition, brief summaries of the 16 afternoon workshops are included so that the reader may share the flavor of those participatory sessions as well. In the workshops, techniques such as role playing, simulation, panel minipresentations, and the hard-nosed question and answer method were used to stimulate participation and to motivate thinking.

As an additional outcome of this project, the Consumer Commission on the Accreditation of Health Services, Inc. has written a manual[1] for consumers serving on health care decision-making bodies. This manual will assist consumers who must systematically examine and gather information about medical technology so that they can make informed decisions.

Since 1972, the Consumer Commission on the Accreditation of Health Services, Inc. has been involved in research and information services for consumers in New York City and elsewhere. This conference series was a natural outgrowth of the Consumer Commission's activities in assisting consumers to better understand and assess health care issues.

It is hoped that through the publication of this book, people will begin to think about the issues raised by advances in medical technology. With this information, consumers will be able to take an ever more responsible role in deciding how and for whom the health care system should be operated.

ADS

DR

SBF

June 1979

Reference

1. Frost, S. B., Fearon, Z. & Hyman, H. H. *A consumer's guide to evaluating medical technology.* New York: Consumer Commission on the Accreditation of Health Services Inc., 1979.

PROJECT ADVISORY COMMITTEE FOR THE NATIONAL SCIENCE FOUNDATION CONFERENCES*

DONALD RUBIN, Co-Chairperson
ALLEN D. SPIEGEL, Ph.D., Co-Chairperson

Alan P. Brownstein	Community Service Society, New York, N.Y.
Bernard Challenor, M.D.	Columbia University College of Physicians and Surgeons, New York, N.Y.
Marshall England	New York City Health Systems Agency Board
Frank Grad	Columbia University Law School, New York, N.Y.
Herbert H. Hyman, Ph.D.	Hunter College, New York, N.Y.
Sylvia Law, J.D.	New York University Law School
Arthur Levin	Center for Medical Consumers and Health Care Information, New York, N.Y.
Louis Levine	Group Health Inc., New York, N.Y.
Sidney Lew	United Fund of Greater New York
Al Lopez	Community Advisory Board, Metropolitan Hospital, New York, N.Y.
Malcom McKay	New York Life Insurance Co.
Barbara Mercado	Committee for a National Health Service Board, New York, N.Y.
Inder Persaud	Cumberland Hospital, Brooklyn, N.Y.
Lillian Roberts	District Council 37, American Federation of State, County and Municipal Employees (AFSCME), New York

*Affiliations as of the conferences.

George Rothman	United Furniture Workers Insurance Fund, New York, N.Y.
Joan Saltzman	Community Advocates, Inc., New York, N.Y.
Al Smoke	New York City Consumer Assembly
Michael M. Stewart, M.D.	Columbia University College of Physicians and Surgeons, New York, N.Y.
Philip Strax, M.D.	Guttman Institute, New York, N.Y.
Milton Terris, M.D.	New York Medical College
Pedro Velez	Elmhurst Hospital, Queens, N.Y.
Judith B. Wessler	MFY Legal Services, New York, N.Y.
Melvin Yahr, M.D.	Mt. Sinai School of Medicine, New York, N.Y.

Project Staff

Shelley B. Frost	Project Director
Zita Fearon	Research Associate
Ellen Goldensohn	Research Assistant
Jeff Draisin	Research Assistant
Jane Gluckmann	Secretary

CONFERENCE PARTICIPANTS*

Presentors and Moderators—Morning Sessions

David Banta, M.D.	Office of Technology Assessment, Washington, D.C.
Ted Bogue	Public Citizen Health Research Group, Washington, D.C.
Alan P. Brownstein	Community Service Society, New York, N.Y.
Joel N. Buxbaum, M.D.	New York University Medical School, New York, N.Y.
Louis R. M. Del Guercio, M.D.	New York Medical College
Florence B. Fiori, Dr. P.H.	Region II, DHEW, New York
H. Jack Geiger, M.D.	Center for Biomedical Education, City University of New York
Frank C. Giarrizzo	Association of Health Care Consumers, Chicago, Ill.
Gilbert Hollander	New York City Health Systems Agency
John L. S. Holloman, M.D.	Health and Hospitals Corporation of New York City (formerly)
Herbert H. Hyman, Ph.D.	Hunter College, New York, N.Y.
Arthur Levin	Center for Medical Consumers and Health Care Information, New York, N.Y.
Louis L. Levine	Group Health Inc., New York, N.Y.
Harold L. Light	Long Island College Hospital, Brooklyn, N.Y.
Charlotte Muller, Ph.D.	Center for Social Research, City University of New York
Peter Rogatz, M.D.	Rogatz & Myers Associates, New York, N.Y.
Donald Rubin	Consumer Commission on the Accreditation of Health Services, Inc., New York, N.Y.
Herbert Semmel	Consumer Coalition for Health, Washington, D.C.

*Affiliation as of the conferences.

Michael M. Stewart, M.D.	Columbia University College of Physicians and Surgeons, New York, N.Y.
Milton Terris, M.D.	New York Medical College

Afternoon Workshop Panelists

Geraldine Alpert, Ph.D.	New York City Health Systems Agency
Mary Batten	Prenatal Diagnostic Laboratory of New York City
Clyde Behney	Office of Technology Assessment, Washington, D.C.
John Boland, M.D.	Mt. Sinai School of Medicine, New York, N.Y.
Ron Brooke	Brookdale Center on Aging, Hunter College, New York, N.Y.
Andrea Eagan	HealthRight, New York, N.Y.
Marshall England	New York City Health Systems Agency Board
Zita Fearon	Consumer Council to the New York City Health Department
Lawrence Feiner, Ph.D.	Health Care Consultant, New York, N.Y.
Sarah Frierson	New York City Health Systems Agency
Michael Gansl	Health and Hospitals Corporation, New York, N.Y.
Louis R. Gary	Hunter College, New York, N.Y.
Joani George	New York City Health Systems Agency
Edward Gluckmann	Consumer Commission on the Accreditation of Health Services, Inc., New York, N.Y.
Allan Goldstein, M.D.	New York City Health Systems Agency

Norma J. Goodwin, M.D.	Amron Management Consultants, Inc., New York, N.Y.
Enoch Gordis, M.D.	Mt. Sinai School of Medicine, New York, N.Y.
Gail Gordon	Committee for A National Health Service, New York, N.Y.
Frank Grad	Columbia University Law School, New York, N.Y.
Arnold Haber	New York Health Systems Agency, Queens, N.Y.
Doris Haire	American Foundation for Maternal and Child Health, Inc., New York, N.Y.
Neil Heyman	New York City Health Systems Agency, Queens, N.Y.
Kathleen Hunt	New York City Emergency Medical Services System
Marsha Hurst, Ph.D.	Maternity Center Association, New York, N.Y.
Rene Jahiel, M.D.	New York University Medical Center
Michelle Kahmi	Maternity Center Association, New York, N.Y.
Phyllis Klass	New York Hospital, Cornell Medical Center, New York, N.Y.
Sylvia Law, J.D.	New York University Law School
Henry Patrick Leis, Jr., M.D.	New York Medical College
Joseph Levi	Long Island Jewish – Hillside Medical Center, New York, N.Y.
Marvin Lieberman, Ph.D.	New York Academy of Medicine
James Lomax, M.D.	Brookdale Medical Center, Brooklyn, N.Y.
Ruth Watson Lubic	Maternity Center Association, New York, N.Y.
Anthony Mangiaracina	W. R. Grace and Co., New York, N.Y.
Bruce Mansdorf	New York State Health Planning and Development Agency, Albany, N.Y.

Shirley Mayer, M.D.	New York City Health Department
Michael McCann, Ph.D.	Center for Occupational Hazards, New York, N.Y.
Thomas Miller	New York Health Systems Agency, Brooklyn, N.Y.
Eileen Muller	New York City Health Systems Agency
Lois Nadler	New York City Health Systems Agency
Deborah Nagin	New York City Health Systems Agency
Major Karl Nelson	Booth Memorial Medical Center, Queens, N.Y.
Lloyd Novick, M.D.	New York City Health Department
Emil Pascarelli, M.D.	Beekman Downtown Hospital, New York, N.Y.
Nelly Peissachowitz	National Citizens Committee on Nursing Home Reform, New York, N.Y.
Marcia Pinkett-Heller	Columbia University School of Public Health, New York, N.Y.
Benjamin Riskin	Formerly of ERM Health Center, New York, N.Y.
Guy Robbins, M.D.	Memorial Sloan-Kettering Cancer Institute, New York, N.Y.
Mary Robinson	New York City Health Systems Agency, Bronx, N.Y.
Oscar Rosenfeld	New York University School of Social Work, New York, N.Y.
Donald Rubin	Consumer Commission on the Accreditation of Health Services, New York, N.Y.
Paul Sayegh	Civic Action Group of Cobble Hill, Brooklyn, N.Y.
Eugene Sibery	Blue Cross-Blue Shield of Greater New York

David W. Smith, J.D.	New York City Health Systems Agency
Allen D. Spiegel, Ph.D.	Downstate Medical Center, Brooklyn, N.Y.
John Steen	New York Health Systems Agency, Staten Island, N.Y.
Philip Strax, M.D.	New York Medical College
Henry Velez, M.D.	Mt. Sinai Hospital, New York, N.Y.
Judith B. Wessler	MFY Legal Services, New York, N.Y.
William H. White	New York City Health Systems Agency, Brooklyn, N.Y.
William Wolarsky, M.D.	Daughters of Jacob Geriatric Center, Bronx, N.Y.
Catherine Wynkoop	New York City Health Systems Agency
Donna Ganzer Yedvab	Statistical Consultant, New York, N.Y.

Chapter 1

A CONSUMER'S PRIMER ON MEDICAL TECHNOLOGY

Allen D. Spiegel

TECHNOLOGY—A HOUSEHOLD OCCURRENCE

Most people accept the advances of modern technology as a routine part of everyday living despite the wonder and awe that the innovations inspire. Compare the first, elementary aircraft that the Wright brothers flew in 1903 to the jumbo jets that cross continents in a matter of hours; or the difference between riding in a vintage Model T Ford and relaxing in the current upholstered version with air conditioning and four stereo speakers as you travel on smooth highways. Think of all the household appliances and gadgets that make use of plastic and other lightweight newly synthesized materials to allow for easy mobility and reduce the time required for chores.

Yet these wonderous advances come with unintended side effects that may cause harm to the consumer. Jet aircraft pollute the atmosphere and the noise may result in impaired hearing; automobiles spread noxious fumes in the streets and also create a national problem due to death and disability from accidents; during the production of some plastic materials, workers in the factory may develop a form of bladder cancer in the process.

In most cases, the consumer had little or no involvement in the decisions relative to the advances of modern technology. Consumers did not make policy decisions on the construction of jet aircraft, the design of the automobile, or manufacturing the plastic container. Industrial leaders and sometimes government agencies proceeded on their own to make the vital decisions. However, as discovered later, those decisions directly affected the health of the consumer.

Recent events illustrate the direct link of medical technology to the consumer. When the swine flu vaccine was developed and a nationwide immunization program started, some people receiving the vaccine developed a paralytic condition. Surgeons developed the coronary bypass operation to reduce the threat of a heart attack until colleagues began questioning the effectiveness of the procedure. Nuclear power plants produced lower cost energy with reassurances of the safety and efficacy by all concerned, until there was a radiation hazard at the Three Mile Island plant in Pennsylvania. There are many more examples. All the incidents merely serve to reinforce the need for consumers to heed their own counsel regarding technology and their own health.

To bring the examination of technology to the field of health care, this chapter will undertake the following:

- Note useful baseline technological definitions
- Examine the values of consumers and providers that influence the advances of technology
- Review the organizational mechanisms by which technology enters the health care delivery system
- Describe the assessment of medical technology with emphasis on safety and efficacy of innovations
- Detail roles for consumers to play in the medical technology process
- Note recommendations for improving the consumer's role in the health care delivery system

A number of the points made in this chapter will be echoed by others in this book. These points are worth repeating and should assist in getting the concepts across. In addition, the references listed at the end of the chapter provide a beginning for those who wish to further pursue the subject of medical technology and the consumer.

Despite the fact that the threats of medical technology have received a great deal of attention in the mass media, the benefits have also been bountiful. Consumers are being placed in positions where they must weigh the costs and benefits. A variety of methods of examining the issues will be presented here.

USEFUL TECHNOLOGICAL DEFINITIONS AND CONCEPTS

In general, medical technology refers to the drugs, devices, and medical and surgical procedures used in medical care, and the organizational and supportive systems within which such care is provided. Conceptually, technological innovations consist of two parts: an idea and the end product that eventually evolves. However, it is possible to be innovative in the creation of ideas without following through to the production of an end product. This could be the so-called idea man. Most likely, medical technology would consist of both the idea and the end product.[1]

In addition, medical technology can be classified according to the intended use of the end product. Two categories of technology exist: mechanical medical purposes and those affecting the individual's body.[2]

Mechanical medical purposes include

1. Diagnostic technologies that assist in determining what disease processes are occurring in a patient, e.g., automated laboratory testing

2. Preventive technologies that protect individuals from disease, e.g., vaccinations
3. Therapeutic or rehabilitative technologies that relieve individuals from disease and its effects, e.g., whirlpool baths
4. Organizational and administrative technologies used to deliver health care as effectively as possible, e.g., mobile vans as treatment centers
5. Supportive technologies used to provide patients with needed services such as hospital beds and food services

Physical medical purposes include

1. Techniques applied to a patient by a health care provider using skills and/or knowledge, e.g., medical history taking and diagnosis
2. Drugs applied to, ingested by, or injected into humans to prevent, treat, or diagnose disease or other medical conditions
3. Devices, ranging from small instruments to major machines, used in medical care, e.g., electric thermometer to CAT scanner
4. Procedures involving a combination of provider skills with drugs and/or devices that could be quite complex in the therapeutic process

Thus, medical technology can begin with an idea that leads to the development of some end product that can be classified as mechanical in nature or having a physical application. Following this, the medical technology can be regarded as complex or sophisticated. *Sophisticated medical technology* refers to situations where the new intervention is able to eliminate the disease and restores the patient to his prior health condition. In addition, sophisticated technology could be preventive and effectively block the factors that cause the disease and/or conditions in the first place. Polio vaccine would be an example. *Complex medical technology,* sometimes called half-way technology, uses techniques and devices that alleviate the conditions but do not eliminate the disease state. This complex technology is often more costly than sophisticated technology. Kidney dialysis is a complex medical technology that involves intricate machines and complicated techniques to help the patient to live but does not eliminate the disease state.[3]

Another phrase that will be heard often in discussions is *technologic imperative.* This refers to an attitude that stimulates the development and use of medical technology at a rapid rate. This occurs when both health care providers and the public feel a compulsion to use the latest techniques, the newest drugs, and the most complex devices. This takes place regardless of the technology's improved ability to combat a particular condition or disease.

Critics accuse the American health care provider of "overdoctoring" and "overmedicating" the population to the detriment of the people. Regardless of size, hospitals desire the status that comes from following the technologic imperative. Consumers likewise secure gratification from knowing that their doctors prescribe the newest drug and use the most up-to-date equipment.

If the technologic imperative is to be curbed, there must be an adequate assessment of medical technology. As with any evaluative procedures, there are problems of bias and limitations. This involves *technology assessment,* a comprehensive form of policy research that examines the short- and long-term social consequences of the application or use of technology. It is an analysis of social rather than technical issues, and is especially concerned with unintended, indirect, or delayed social impacts.[4] It can also be defined as an effort to examine the benefits, costs, and risks of a technology or technologic development in a rigorous manner as a step in the process of determining what, if any, governmental action may be necessary or desirable to direct the development or use of the technology along lines which will achieve an optimization of the benefit-cost/risk ratio.[5]

Since the word efficacy was used, it is worthwhile to look

at some definitions from various sources. Safety and efficacy are the two words most often used relative to the acceptance of medical technology. Safety is rather well understood and means that no harm shall be done to the patient. Efficacy is a bit more problematic. Table 1-1 gives brief definitions from the Food, Drug and Cosmetic Act, the World Health Organization, the federal Office of Technology Assessment, a health care dictionary, and from a leading researcher.

VALUES AND ATTITUDES OF PROVIDERS OF MEDICAL TECHNOLOGY

The values and attitudes held by health care providers and by consumers are of strategic importance in the development and application of medical technologies. At times, these values are not consistent and may even be in conflict. Values may also waver depending upon whether the medical technology is applied to yourself or to others and with a consideration of the state of the art of the intended medical technology.

Consumers have often said, "If we can send a man to the moon, why can't we find a cure for cancer?" Some other ending can be tagged to the "why can't we" phrase to suit personal interests. On the other hand, there are those who say that certain medical innovations cause more illness than they cure. Thus, an immediate value conflict is identified. One consumer viewpoint is expressed in the slogan of the Sierra Club, a consumer group interested in the protection of the environment, "We are not blindly against scientific and technical progress, but we are against blind scientific and technical progress."[7]

Yet, the possibility of easing human suffering caused by disease is a most compelling motivation to many researchers. In fact, these people may be completely committed zealots of their cause holding the noblest values. There is a great tendency in the health care field, perhaps more than in any other, to keep doing something and not to just stand still. Frustration can be

Table 1–1 Selected Definitions of "Efficacy"[6]

Source	*Term defined*	*Definition*
Federal Food, Drug, and Cosmetic Act*	Effectiveness, Efficacy (interchangeable)	A drug is effective if it has "the effect it purports or is represented to have under the conditions of use prescribed, recommended, or suggested in the proposed labeling thereof"
A. Cochrane†	Efficacy (interchangeable with effectiveness)	"The effect of a particular medical action in altering the natural history of a particular disease for the better"
World Health Organization‡	Efficacy	Benefit or utility to the individual of the service, treatment regimen, drug, preventive or control measure advocated or applied
Discursive Dictionary of Health Care §	Efficacy (as a variant of effectiveness)	"The degree to which diagnostic, preventive, therapeutic, or other action or actions (undertaken under ideal circumstances) achieves the desired result"
Office of Technology Assessment‖	Efficacy	The probability of benefit to individuals in a defined population from a medical technology applied for a given medical problem under ideal conditions of use

* USDHEW, Food and Drug Administration. *Code of Federal Regulations, Title 21.* Washington, D.C.: Govt. Printing Office, 1977.
† Cochrane, A. *Effectiveness and efficiency*. London: Burgess and Son Ltd., 1972.
‡ World Health Organization. *Statistical indicators for the planning and evaluation of public health programmes.* Geneva: WHO Technical Report series No. 472. 1971.
§ U.S. Congress, House Committee on Interstate and Foreign Commerce. *A discursive dictionary of health care.* Washington, D.C.: Govt. Printing Office, 1976.
‖ Office of Technology Assessment. *Assessing the efficacy and safety of medical technologies.* Washington, D.C.: Govt. Printing Office, 1978.

emotionally overwhelming if a health care provider has to stand by and do nothing while the patient obviously needs help. Help is often attempted even if the real value is unknown.

It is worthwhile noting that medicine began essentially as a social science. Few, if any, effective medical technologies existed prior to the scientific revolution of the 1800s. Physicians practiced the *art* of medicine rather than the *science* of medicine. Hands were held, brows were wiped, soft words were spoken, prayers were rendered, and house calls were common. Perhaps the past 50 or 75 years really accounted for the giant technologic strides foward. With that foward movement came the changes in values. People wanted the prescription for the new miracle drug; equipment to poke and probe, and after analysis, to yield a definitive diagnosis had to be better than the old way. Bigger is better and biggest is the best. Now, values are shifting again and the following quote illustrates a patient's viewpoint:[8]

> The patient sees all this (the present health care system) differently from any of us (health professionals). He sees it from the viewpoint of one who spends an interminable amount of time with a professional who is overworked, overpaid, delivers his comments with a bit of arrogance, sees the patient as an illness or a diseased organ and has no concept of or interest in the patient as a total person, who, among other things, is paying a hundred dollars a day for room and board which is not nearly so comfortable as the room he could get at the Holiday Inn for a third of that.

The following is an illustration of the depersonalization that has been accepted by most patients as a necessary evil associated with the sophisticated care and the technological advances.[9]

> *Medical Science and Things*
>
> The doctor-thing is his white coat unhesitatingly pushed open the door of the hospital room. The door had no lock or latch so

that he needed only to push it and felt no need to knock. It was a "semi-private" room, so that the doctor looked from the one "semi-private" to the other, wondering which was his. Finally, the white-coated doctor ask with a rising inflection, "Mr. . . .?" The semi-private sitting on the far bed, as if afraid to muss it, was in a new bathrobe and stiff slippers. The far-bed, semi-private replied with a rising inflection,"Yes?". In his white coat, the doctor-thing said, "I'm Doctor . . .." The patient knew, really knew, that this doctor-thing was truly a man of science. "His" doctor had sent him to "the" doctor.

The doctor-thing, still standing, surveyed the patient-thing with a practiced eye. The patient-thing quickly, even embarrassingly, crushed out his half-smoked cigarette. "What's the trouble?", asked the doctor-thing.

"I have a feeling here."

The doctor-thing pulled up a chair and sat. "Point to it", he directed. "About here", said the patient-thing. "How long?", "How often?", "Nature of?", "Radiates to?", "Brought on by?", "Relieved by?", "Pain or ache?", "Previous illness?", "Married?", "Children?", "Smoke?", "Drink?", "Job?", "Lie down, please so I can examine you." "Hmm, need some tests." "We'll do a cholecystogram tomorrow, a barium enema next day."

The doctor-thing got up to go. "Waa—what do you think it is?", asked the patient-thing.

"Need the tests to tell."

"But Doctor, what do you—anything serious?"

"We're getting the tests."

The doctor-thing strode out of the "semi-private" room, leaving the door, without a lock or latch, open.*

Yet some professionals argue that the current environment of suspicion of technology and the emphasis on consumer protection may be harmful. One physician contended that if contemporary consumer attitudes had prevailed 20 years ago, artificial heart valve prostheses would never have been developed. Furthermore, the author felt that passage of the Medical Device Amendments Act of 1976 (p.1. 94–295) will make future medical advances extremely difficult. In concluding, the

*W.A. Steiger, "Medical Science and Things," *Health and Human Behavior, 4*(1): 39, Spring 1964.

author calls for someone to protect patients from their so-called protectors.[10]

Another confusing issue is inflationary health care costs. In the consideration of health care costs, two opposing attitudes have emerged relative to medical technology. One view holds that medical technology has been responsible for many advances in the quality and quantity of care as well as for a reduction in death, disability, discomfort, and disease. Even greater strides are projected in the future. An opposing view contends that much of the medical technology development has been ineffective and actually has detracted from the health of the population by using limited dollars that might have been expended in more effective ways to improve health status. Obviously, decisions must be made to accommodate these viewpoints and allow for a rational movement within the health care delivery system. How much investment in technology is warranted? An easy answer is not forthcoming. Resolution will be related to what value society places on the positive and negative answers to the following propositions:

> Increased or sustained funding of biomedical research will yield new or improved technologies to control major health problems.
>
> Viable alternative funding activities can impact on the factors affecting health.
>
> Social, economic, ethical, and political costs and benefits of the first two premises in any combination will be acceptable.
>
> Other social needs competing for limited available resources will be satisfied.
>
> Social and ethical concerns about the availability of life-saving, life-prolonging, and life-enhancing technologies will be resolved to the satisfaction of both consumer and provider.[11]

While society and individuals have to consider these premises, the Department of Health, Education and Welfare commented that the health industry is highly technology-dependent and much of its increasing technologic base stems from biomedical research. Yet, the direction of medical technology appears to respond to individual values that desire technologies for treatment of specific ailments. Unfortunately, few people have values that call for technology for the betterment of the entire society. Private interests usually prevail.

In view of the causal relationships that exist between illness and specific variables, the following attitudinal stances should be examined for an estimation of where they fit in the value systems of consumers and providers:

> Today's major health problems may be more amenable to preventive interventions and more cost-effective.
>
> Health problems may be more effectively controlled by stressing measures aimed at the population rather than providing one-to-one treatment services.
>
> Despite the attention to prevention and to population strategies, environmental factors have to allow individuals to live healthier lives.[12]

In a discussion of policies on food additives and drugs, a report of the National Academy of Sciences asks "How safe is safe?" A very real sense of problems faced by consumers and others in their decision making and their value considerations is presented. Difficulties are numerous and raise more issues for research than answers.[13]

HEW's *Forward Plan for Health* notes that:[14]

> There exists a wide spectrum of views on the potential usefulness of technology and research in health care, i.e., from that of providing most of the answers to our health care problems, to

> that of having a questionable impact and an attendant progressive dehumanization of the system. It has been demonstrated that technology can significantly affect development of new products, health service capacity and quality, communications, data processing and storage, utilization of allied health personnel and other important areas of the health field. Further progress must build upon these advances in health care technology through more effective relationships among the principal segments—universities, hospitals and medical centers, private industry and other elements of the private sector, and government.

Thus, the values and attitudes of consumers and providers reflect some of the thinking illustrated earlier. However, at this time the values of consumers are taking on more weight than ever before. Previously, health care providers held their own values and paternally accepted the consumer values in their decision making. Now, the consumer is a legal part of the decision-making process and the consumer values have to be considered in the same context as those of the provider. It is no longer acceptable that "poppa knows best." An Advisory Committee on Industrial Innovation appointed a public interest subcommittee to make recommendations on policy alternatives. This subcommittee concluded that, "government has both a moral and legal responsibility to promote innovations of a type that will further the goals of our society and will fulfill the basic social and human needs of its citizens."[15]

Organizational Patterns, Medical Technology, and the Health Care Delivery System

From an organizational viewpoint, medical technology has to be considered relative to the aspect of the health care delivery system being affected. Once that is determined, planners can proceed with figuring out the organization required to carry out the technological goals. Various schemes have been proposed to break down the organizational components as listed below with some indication of technology that is involved:[16,17]

Administrative: Electronics equipment used to schedule admissions, to analyze laboratory samples, to enter data into medical records, and to be an integral part of a multiphasic testing activity.

Clinical: Equipment to do surgery using microscopes, to use organ transplants, for dialysis and to install pacemakers.

Pharmaceutical: Computerized distribution of drugs and simulated testing devices.

Repair: Mainly dealing with surgical devices replacing worn out or damaged human anatomical parts.

Hardware: Physical plant and equipment items such as microwave ovens and solar heating units.

This framework allows planners to consider the patient population that may be involved, the professional manpower needs, the training required for workers, the unit costs as well as the overall financial capability. Key elements can be identified for each of the varying categories of technology and these elements can form a check list for decision makers. For example, administrative technology would involve management types as opposed to a repair technology which may involve mainly surgical professionals.

Regardless of the technology, experience has indicated that the impact of the technology is characterized by the following three processes:

1. Due to the alternatives, the decision making will be diffused.
2. Part of the decision making will be relinquished to others in the health care system.
3. There will be a shift of some of the decision making to the object of the decision, the patient.[18]

These characteristics are fairly obvious and related directly to the increasing sophistication of medical technology.

With more alternatives, the decisions will involve many others and will be diffused and given to other specialties. With the patient being given the opportunity to choose, the individual may make the final choice of providing his or her warm body for the procedure.

Evolution of the Medical Care System

Since this section deals with the organization of medicine, it might be useful to consider the evolution of the present health care delivery system. Again, each of the components carries with it an organizational system that relates to all the other elements. For example, the education of professionals results in a direct one-to-one impact on how they organize themselves to deliver care once they begin to practice in their private office, in the hospital, or in any other health care facility. This evolution of a modern medical care system can be summarized as the following:

Incorporation of scientific principles and methods into the medical practice of the late 19th and early 20th centuries.

As a result of the growing scientific base, technology was refined stressing chemotherapeutic and surgical procedures.

Responding to the available technology, medical education emphasized those technical skills required for the diagnosis and treatment of patients upon whom the technology could be applied.

Emergence of a host of highly skilled and competent practitioners from the educational institutions to use the available technology.

To spread the use of the new technology, a considerable amount of capital was invested in facilities and equipment.

Development, in a reciprocal fashion, of the world's largest biomedical research community through the National Institutes of Health.

Through that research, the development and subsequent application of a host of therapeutic technologies.

Based on this technology, the creation of an elaborate medical care delivery system to pass along to patients the fruits of the technology.

Growth of both public and private marketing and funding mechanisms to stimulate and facilitate the use of available services.[19]

A review of this evolutionary system will certainly tend to indicate the circular motion of the components in the medical care system. Some may even call the system a "catch-22." Obviously, many of the features of the medical care system are linked to the inherent values placed upon technology by both professionals and consumers. Some consumers do not consider their physician to be good unless they get a prescription before leaving the office, whether or not they really need it. Some health care providers believe that they cannot practice medicine unless the newest and best piece of machinery is being used in the office. With both parties in the physician–patient encounter placing a premium on the application of medical technology, it will be difficult to change the direction of the evolutionary stream unless the values also show a corresponding change.

Organizational Steps in Medical Innovation

Within this evolutionary model of the medical care system, a logical, linear sequence is included for the development, diffusion, and use of medical technologies. Highlighted in this sequence is the fact that it is usually possible to identify a medical innovation prior to widespread application. This means that the innovation can be tested for efficacy and safety. However, everybody knows that life does not move in logical and linear steps and variances occur with regularity. In fact, a well known law states, "If anything can go wrong in research, it will." Nevertheless, the process is noted below with the seven most common steps in the innovation sequence:

1. Research yields new knowledge to relate to the existing data base.
2. Applied research translates new knowledge into new technology and sets into action a strategy to move the technology into the health care delivery system.
3. Controlled clinical trials or other means evaluate the safety and efficacy of the new technology.
4. Demonstration and control programs indicate the feasibility for widespread use.
5. Diffusion of the technology into medical practice takes place through continuing trials and demonstrations and acceptance in the professional community.
6. Integration into the educational curriculum of professionals and into the general education of the lay community takes place largely through mass media.
7. Routine skillful and balanced use of the new developments in the health care delivery system results.[20]

Of course, governmental regulations and controls are interwoven into the sequence such as requirements of the federal Food and Drug Administration for several levels of research and testing to prove safety and efficacy. Again, consumers should be aware that safety was a longer standing requirement than efficacy. Drugs were only required to demonstrate efficacy as the result of federal legislation passed in the 1960s after the world-wide Thalidomide incident triggered a congressional committee into action. In fact, government agencies now rank some items according to their efficacy as "helpful," "probably effective," "ineffective," or "limited effectiveness." Many over-the-counter items fall into the least effective classifications.

Other commentators have also noted that the development of medical technology usually adds the following characteristics:

Development processes occur over a long period of time.

These processes are typically international in character involving individuals and institutions in several countries.

Medical technology innovations may draw upon technical developments in areas outside of medicine.

Several developmental processes may interact in various ways as alternative approaches are considered.

It is probable that a cadre of physicians will collect around a given technology laying the groundwork for further development.[21]

If this developmental model is correct, consumers have a difficult task in the exercise of their decision-making powers. Consumers must keep getting information over protracted periods of time. They may need to maintain files and storage cabinets to retrieve the material when needed. If the technology is international, there could be a need for translations, for expenses for postage and for expert help in locating the foreign researchers and institutions. When medical technology relates to the general advance in technical ability, the consumer will be hard put to locate information easily from the commercial market. If the cadre of researchers acts protectively regarding their innovation, it will be difficult for a lay person to crack the hard exterior and get accurate understandable information. With these caveats in mind, the concept of an organized independent consumer network to supply data takes on even more meaning.

Health Status and Technological Accomplishments

Continuing on from the evolution of the medical care system with an explanation of the innovation sequence and the characteristics of technological advancement, we come to a listing of the accomplishments of a medical care system with a heavy emphasis on technology. These accomplishments include:

Accumulation of an impressive body of knowledge gained through research.

Scientifically based tools and techniques that are used by scores of highly trained and qualified health care providers.

An increase in longevity through control of infectious disease and reduced mortality among infants and children.

Effective treatment of accidental trauma.

Sociomedical programs such as the maternal and child health activities and the community mental health centers.

Contributions of public health programs to the quality of life.

Provision of counseling and caring to many patients.[22]

Again, the consumer may be impressed with the accomplishments and may agree that, as a nation, we are healthier than ever. Yet, time after time accomplishments related to technological advances have been refuted by investigators who claim that the trend was moving in that direction anyhow. This disagreement has not been settled. Consumers should be aware of the differences.

Role of Executives

Now that some attention has been given to the administrative aspects of the organizational patterns of medical technology development, it is time to consider the role of the influential executives in the health care system. Physicians, in particular, and health care providers, in general, hold that following the technologic imperative results in better quality care. This means that more technology and more use of medical advances is better just because there is more of it. Thinking of this nature is stressed during the professional's training and during practical experiences with patients. A noted economist commented "in health care one has the strong impression that one of the reasons for rising health care costs has been the proclivity of doctors and hospitals to adopt any plausible new thing—drugs, surgical methods, equipment—that increases capability in any dimension without regard to cost."[23] To further aggravate this problem, it seems that efforts to control the purchase of new unwarranted equipment are failing. Reviewers noted that, despite controls such as certificate of need, more than 90 percent of applications are approved.[24] Even if there were more stringent controls, there is some doubt that rising costs would be severly curtailed since equipment purchases may only account for 9 percent of total hospital inflation.[25]

Decision-Making Techniques

So, how are decisions to be made? Decision makers must develop structured procedures to evaluate alternative choices. In talking about hospitals learning to do more with less, gracefully, one author urged the input of a broad range of people into the decision. He stated that the consensus approach was worth the time and effort.[26] To establish a baseline for consumers, the following definitions of decision-making techniques are briefly noted:

Operations Research/Management Science. This is the systematic use of quantitative methods, techniques, and tools to the analysis of problems involving the operation of [man-machine] systems.

Cost-Benefit Analysis. This is a practical way to express the costs and benefits in terms of dollars by placing values on all aspects of the projects.

Zero-Base Budgeting. This technique examines the base for all existing programs taking nothing for granted. After the review, all the projects are ranked from lower to higher priority activities.

Systems Analysis. This method takes a wholistic view of an entire system and evaluates objectives and alternatives in an analytic fashion to determine the consequences.

Policy Analysis. This method is similar to systems analysis with more stress on political and organizational considerations.[27]

While consumers may be acquainted with the various decision-making techniques, it is obvious that the professionals will have more resources to carry out the actual processes. Furthermore, the health care providers may have expert personnel on their staffs to assist them. In any event, consumers will be very hard pressed to use these decision-making tools without the assistance of health planning staffs or others. Importantly, the consumers should know that these tools are used in varying ways and there is no consensus upon which tool is the best to use in which situation. Of course, different tools may yield different results depending upon the objective of the person using that particular decision-making technique.

Organizational Motivation—Public or Private?

Can consumers accept the idea that medical technology is developed by men and women of good will and high ideals?

After all, scientific training and the Hippocratic Oath, among others, all emphasize that the physician shall do no harm to his patients. Consider the following quotation:[28]

> I have had the feeling for a long time that in health care we keep attacking the wrong villain. Technology really isn't the villain; it's the end-stage, the distribution system, that's out of control. The problem is that there are things lying around for which there is still reimbursement, even though medical practitioners long ago said that they don't make any sense. The question is can we change this without killing off the nonvillain—technology?

Obviously, the prospect of achieving an improvement in patient health status is overwhelmingly motivational in specific cases. In those instances, the consumer accepts the good will idea without reservation. In writing about the first person to agree to a heart transplant, it was noted that people thought that Mr. Washkansky was brave to make that decision. However, the surgeon commented:[29]

> For a dying man, it is not a difficult decision because he knows he is at the end. If a lion chases you to the bank of a river filled with crocodiles, you will leap into the water convinced you have a chance to swin to the other side. But you would never accept such odds if there was no lion.

Consumers sitting on agencies where decisions have to be made will be put into the predicament of evaluating proposals from individual as well as the community viewpoints. As illustrated by the quotes above, this will be difficult.

A Futuristic Health Care Organization

To move the technology concept into the future, one author proposed a cybernated health care system in an article entitled, "Goodbye Dr. Welby."[30] He assumes that by the beginning of the 21st century medical technicians and allied health professionals will usurp those tasks currently performed by physicians, who will become obsolete. Six steps in the standard routine of a physician will be cybernated as follows:

1. A computer will take the medical history from the patient.
2. Machines will perform the physiological tests such as the recording of blood pressure and heart sounds.
3. A computer then takes the data from steps one and two, analyzes the results, and orders any additional tests.
4. Data from steps one, two, and three are then analyzed by the computer which comes forth with a probable diagnosis and suggested treatments.
5. Treatment is implemented by allied health personnel and technicians.
6. Computer prepares a prognosis which is given in mathematical terms.

As an organizational pattern, this scheme uses a high technologic approach. Will it be acceptable to consumers and professionals? Currently, consumers may have difficulty with the relinquishing of the human aspects of medical care despite the obvious intent to deliver the highest quality of care. In the decision-making process, consumers should register their doubts and seek out changes in the organizational patterns to make the technology conform to their concepts of patients as people. Consumers must be careful to avoid outcomes where, as one author noted, people will "become more and more the bewildered dependents on inaccessible castles wherein inscrutable technicians conjure with their fate."[31]

Utilization of Medical Technology

In thinking about the organization of medical technology, the question of utilization is uppermost after safety and efficacy. Will the innovation be used by the providers and the consumers? Actually, the consumers agree to allow the provider to use the technology and usually do not have the choice of using the equipment themselves. Recently, the swine flu vaccination program drove this point home. People stopped coming to get the vaccine after the news about the paralytic side effects appeared in the mass media. People did not feel that the danger of swine flu was strong enough to overcome the threat of more serious side effects. Table 1-2 identifies 17 medical technologies that have been evaluated along with brief comments about their current assessment. It is interesting to note some reservations about extremely common procedures such as appendectomy, tonsillectomy, and pap smears. This is the type of information that consumers should be aware of when making decisions that will affect the utilization of medical technologies throughout the community.

On the other hand, it should be noted that some lawyers have written about the possibility of the use of computers raising the risk of malpractice.[32] Their contention was that a health provider's failure to use the computer when it could have cured, minimized, or prevented medical problems may have been medical malpractice. Standards of high quality care were not being followed. This type of thinking can be expanded considerably if any medical technology procedure is substituted for the word computer. Incidentially, computers can already be used in the health care delivery system for the following purposes:

- Computer based consultation to other providers
- Automated medical records such as the Problem Oriented Medical Information System (PROMIS)
- Decision analysis using branching trees
- Simulated clinical cognition using mannequins for training
- Problem-solving consultations in internal medicine via the INTERNIST program[33]

It is the premise of experts in the use of instrumentation in the delivery of health services that the medical profession is

Table 1–2 Current Assessment of 17 Technological Medical Procedures[34]

Procedure	*Assessment*
Pap smear for cervical cancer*	Widely used for more than 30 years with no demonstration of efficacy through a controlled trial.
Amniocentesis	Appears to be safe and efficacious but there are complex ethical and legal issues.
Chicken pox vaccine	Positive benefits are relatively small while potential risks are large.
Mammography†	Widely used before questions about safety were raised to counter claims of efficacy.
Prophylactic oral antibiotics in elective colon surgery	Use is based on surmise, not on results of testing.
Skull x-ray†	Recognizable risks and large financial costs knowns. Appears to be overused technology.
Electronic fetal monitoring‡	Relative efficacy and benefit not established. May be associated with considerable risk and financial costs.
Surgery for coronary artery disease‡	Based on scientific rationale but may be of measureable benefit to some patients.
Tonsillectomy*	Efficacy and indications for use not adequately understood. Available evidence seems to indicate that many unjustified operations are performed.
Appendectomy*	Relative benefits and risks have not been fully evaluated.
Hysterectomy	Efficacious for some conditions. Some consider the operation overused. Most physicians and consumers appear to consider the procedure valuable.
Drug treatment for hypertension	Such treatment clearly indicated and well-designed studies show efficacy.
Drug treatment for otitis media in children	Universally used and with confirmed efficacy of sulfonamides. More expensive antibiotics often prescribed. Decongestants and antihistamines have no demonstrated efficacy.

Table 1–2 Continued

Procedure	*Assessment*
Cast application for forearm fracture	Efficacy and safety are obvious and established by experience in medical settings.
Treatment of Hodgkin's disease	Efficacy and safety well demonstrated by series of well-designed clinical trials.
Chemotherapy for lung cancer	Efficacy is very limited. Drugs and hormones inherently risky and costs are high.
Hyperbaric oxygen treatment for cognitive deficits in elderly	Insurance carriers and Medicare ruled that this treatment is not medically accepted or effective and they will not reimburse for it.

*Not completely assessed for efficacy.
†Diffused rapidly before careful assessment.
‡Concern about risks.

behind in assimilating the advances of technology.[35] Some used to say that it took at least three to five years to move from the new advance to the adoption in routine practice. Perhaps this is somewhat shortened through the communications network in existence today. Yet, others claim that new governmental regulations will expand that time gap and also increase the cost of utilization when that time approaches.

In any event, the question of the appropriate utilization of medical technology is a valid issue for consumers to ponder when they assume their decision-making roles. Of course, a major part of the utilization problem is concerned with the organizational aspects of the health care delivery system.

Effect and Impact of Medical Technology

A major issue for consumers to grapple with relative to the overall organization of the health care delivery system relates to the effect and/or impact of technology on the system. Subtle impacts of medical technology are important beyond the one-to-one use with individuals or in other activities. For example, the microscope was invented in the 1650s, long before the germ theory came into existence. However, this technologic advance paved the way for researchers who began using the device to look at the minute organisms. An economic expert claims that advances in knowledge were the biggest single source of national economic growth from 1929 to 1969.[36] In sum, the effect has to be looked at with a larger scope than merely the treatment of a single person.

Five areas and questions have been posited for evaluation of the effect of technology:

1. Technical capability: Does the device perform reliably and deliver accurate information?
2. Diagnostic accuracy: Does use of the device permit accurate diagnoses?
3. Diagnostic impact: Does use of the device replace other diagnostic procedures including surgical exploration and biopsy?
4. Therapeutic impact: Do results obtained from the device affect planning and delivery of therapy?
5. Patient outcome: Does use of the device contribute to improved health of the patient?[37]

Patient outcome, of course, has the most attraction for the public. This involves the considerations of safety and efficacy and the changes caused by the technology. For example, sulfa drugs, antibiotics, antipsychotic drugs, and vaccines have all contributed to allowing patients to be treated in practitioner's offices rather than in hospitals. These safe and effective technologies appear to have yielded a favorable impact on the health care delivery system. However, the outcome is not always so beneficial. Effectiveness of radical mastectomies for breast cancer are now questioned[38]; coronary care units (CCUs) may not be saving as many lives as purported.[39,40] Questions have been raised regarding the safety and efficacy of oral drug treatment for diabetics,[41,42] respiratory therapy,[43,44] oral decongestants,[45] thermography for diagnosing breat cancer,[46] ergotamine for migraine headache,[47] immune serum globulin for preventing hepatitis,[48] and intensive care for pulmonary edema.[49] While it is true that perfect information on the impact of technology can never be attained, it is equally obvious from the long list of questions regarding safety and efficacy of established technologies that more can be done to improve the evaluation. Consumers with a critical attitude may be able to insist upon more thorough studies of the impact of technologic changes.

Impact on the System from Technology

How has the integration of medical technology into the organized pattern of the health care delivery system altered the nation's health status? What problems are arising? Some implications of the impact can be seen in the following list:

Diseases to be treated within the health care system are changing. Babies saved through improved neonatal care may be blind, brain damaged, or crippled and require a lifetime of social and health services. Elderly people are saved from pneumonia with antibiotics but they "linger on" trying to secure adequate care.

Frequent "medical miracles" raise the expectations of the public when they need care. If people do not get the same care as they saw on television, more malpractice suits may follow.

Use of the new technology itself makes physicians and hospitals more susceptible to law suits if a pacemaker has a malfunction or if equipment develops a mechanical failure.

New issues need answers regarding ethics and priorities. Who gets the limited number of transplant organs? How long shall clinically dead patients receive life support?

Basic primary care has a lower priority than areas where new technology can be used. Caring aspects of medicine are lost among the shiny pieces of hardware.

Complex medical equipment means that there will be more specialization among physicians as well as allied health care personnel. This results in impersonalization in care.

Continuing education takes on more emphasis since professionals need to keep up-to-date. Mandates are appearing in licensing bodies and professional societies requiring that professionals take continuing education courses to maintain membership or their specialty ranking.

Because the equipment is so expensive, physicians have to share the technologies within an institution or group rather than have the equipment available in the office.

Smaller institutions can not afford the expensive equipment and have to refer patients to larger hospitals for services.[50]

While this is a long list, it is not exhaustive. Effects of technology outside of the health care system are also widespread. Consider the education of the handicapped children; the housing for the elderly; the legal system involved in malpractice suits; the manufacturing companies and the employment opportunities. All these other systems also impact on the application of medical technology. All are factors that must be related to the decision-making process.

Costs of Medical Technology

For a long time the cost of medical technology was absorbed without question into the health care system. Both consumers and providers passed along costs that were reimbursed by third-party payers. A majority of consumers had their health insurance partially or wholly paid for by their employers and were protected from the out-of-pocket costs themselves. Those dollars were invisible as far as the family budget was concerned. This type of situation is alien to the more mundane areas of production where input and outcome are closely measured with an eye for a profit at the end of the cycle.

Currently, federal legislation and regulations emphasize the approach of cost containment. Research funds are advertised with that objective. All types of organizational activities are planned to achieve cost reductions. Quality care activities such as Professional Standards Review Organizations (PSROs) are established to review length of hospital stays and the use of specific therapies. In effect, the inflationary costs finally caught up with and passed the desire to get the biggest and the best.

Studies indicate that technology has saved money and raised the cost of medical care. Consumers must be aware that determining the cost of medical care technology is quite difficult. A good deal more research has to be undertaken to positively link the process of health care to outcomes resulting from the care. Most of the existing studies have been concerned with examinations of the caring process and not the outcomes.[51,52] This is the same situation that occurs when the surgery is a success but the patient dies.

Consumers must ask probing questions about how the costs were calculated regarding technologies. There should be logical answers to questions about the total cost of the use of technology and the improvement in the health status of the patient.

Roles for Consumers in the Technology Process

Consumer's Role Enlarged

In most of the references relating to medical technology, there is little or no mention of the consumer/patient or recipient of the technology. Usually, a health care provider stance dominates the material. There are a number of possible reasons for this and some will be pursued here. In any event, Congress has greatly elevated the role of the consumer in decisions regarding medical technology. Section 1503 of P.L. 93–641 states that the National Council on Health Planning and Development

> shall advise, consult with and make recommendations to the Secretary with respect to . . . (3) an evaluation of the implications of new medical technology for the organization, delivery, and equitable distribution of health care services.

In line with this mandated approach another view calls for consumer action as follows:[53]

> I think there ought to be something broader than just government agencies making the decisions about technology. We should use the outside scientists and consumers to make the final decisions. It ought to be the government's responsibility to put before them the evidence in the best way that it can.

Some knowledgeable consumers are going to say that is similar to what exists today. It sounds like token consumer participation. Let's explore this a bit further.

As mentioned earlier, a great majority of new medical technologies enter the system through the reimbursement mechanism. Good and bad alike, the technologies become intertwined in the system without sufficient assessment and are difficult to withdraw once entrenched. Society has few opportunities to actually choose a technology. Choices take place haphazardly through reimbursement, licensing, or authorization.

Who Makes the Decisions?

Consumers usually do not make the technologic decisions. Why? Some possible answers are revealed in the following quotes:

1. To ward off disease or recover health, men as a rule find it easier to depend on the healers than to attempt the more difficult task of living wisely.[54]
2. It seems that the more effective technology is, the less responsibility many consumers exercise with respect to their own health.[55]
3. In the United States, our social objectives are so diffuse as to be meaningless operationally. Such diffuseness thus leaves a great deal of room to maneuver in the bargaining, negotiating, and trade-off process. We are witnessing the emerging political battle of disease caused by our increasing medical technology. The moral then is: pick your favorite disease and lobby.[56]
4. The physician has to be reeducated about the uses of technology. But the government, which is the only body that has the responsibility and the funds available, has been totally oblivious of the fact that you cannot use technology to reduce costs unless both the patient and the physician know how to use the materials. The reason we do not appreciate the cost saving is because the majority of physicians and patients do not know how to use it. There is a desperate need to educate them.[57]

In sum, consumers are happy to have the healers make the decisions, do not particularly take care of their own health, have a wide open political situation in the health care arena, and need an education along with the providers.

Revitalize the Consumer's Role

In view of this pessimistic attitude, how can consumers participate in public policy decisions regarding medical technology? Assuming the consumer projects the public attitude, then the nation's population anticipates that disease is presumptively curable. Further, it is expected that the cure will be aided and abetted by medical technology at its best. Therefore, to vote against new technology is inherently evil. Consumers placed in decision-making positions are then asked to consider approval of technologies rationally and logically. This may go against the grain of the social values of the consumers.

Nevertheless, it is apparent that consumers must move from merely supplying the warm bodies for health care providers to being active, equal participants in the decision-making process. It should not be too much to ask that the technology be proven safe, effective, and worth the cost. Blind faith in experts has not always been shown to be the best route for consumers to take. Recent experiences with nuclear power plants and revelations about the dangers of atomic testing reinforce this viewpoint. Furthermore, callous disregard for anything other than the profit columns by commercial firms also illustrates the consumer's choice dilemma in the detrimental health effects on people living near dumps where industries carelessly tossed their toxic waste materials from the factory.

A major revitalization of the consumer role first requires a considerable strengthening of the critical attitude toward technology. Consumers must play a more vital part and have confidence in their ability to understand plain language. Their lives may depend on this role in the decision-making process.

Recommendations for Improving the Consumer's Role

Based on all the material covered so far and the questions and problems raised repeatedly, several issues stand out as items and areas for suggesting recommendations. These particular problems are presented in the form of questions:

> How can the transfer of new medical technology be facilitated from the research center into the community?
> How can the financial impact of new medical technology be controlled?
> How can the introduction of new medical technology be regulated to avoid harmful side effects?
> How can the emphasis be placed on the development of medical technologies that provide definitive therapy rather than half-way technology?[58]

Again a basic underlying factor emerges when recommendations are to be considered. A recent article noted that the individual should take more responsibility for his own health instead of relying on costly and inefficient medical services. He discussed this point in the reference of the ideology and politics of victim blaming under the title, "You are dangerous to your health." His suggestion noted the difficulty of individualism in a technological age and opted for combining individualism with reformed medicine.[59] An annotated bibliography on consumer participation in health planning adds more on this issue in a number of articles.[60]

Recommendations from Various Sources

To move to specifics, recommendations are quoted from a Citizens Board of Inquiry sponsored by the American Public Health Association. In keeping with the individualistic approach, the report was entitled, "Heal Yourself."[61]

> Health care delivery systems should be organized and made accountable to the public in the following ways:
>
> A. Health professionals should make individual decisions affecting the health of their patients while the public should

become the ultimate determinant of the health care system and of how health care services are delivered, paid for and organized.

B. Consumers must have the dominant role at all levels in the decision-making process of the health care system.

C. While we do not advocate any one particular process to be used in selecting persons to represent consumers in decision-making, the selection process should stress the following principles: 1. The procedure for selecting consumer representatives must be well-known and clear to the community or to the consumer group to which services are being provided; 2. Individual consumers and consumer groups must be able to affect the process of selection; 3. Consumer representatives must be accountable and responsible to the group that they represent.

Consumers must be able to establish goals, objectives and priorities of the newly-structured delivery system and make them effective in the organization and delivery of health services.

A. Adequate resources must be made available to consumer representatives so that they can make appropriate decisions and recommendations. These representatives must become well-informed about the financing, operations and mechanisms of the health care delivery system and their particular part of it. In some cases, consumer representatives will need a professional staff or consultants whose prime responsibility is to consumers and not to the provider mechanism.

B. The power of the consumer to control and influence the delivery system must be exercised at every level of the health care system: facility, service system or program, and neighborhood, city, state, region or nation. This power should include, but not be limited to, making policy, controlling assets (including capital expenditures), facilities, equipment and services. This does not mean that consumers will usurp the doctor's responsibility for meeting his patient's medical needs. On all levels of decision-making, clear lines between policy (the consumer's primary business) and professional judgment regarding the individual patient (the physician's primary business) should be established.

C. Agencies or institutions that render medical services and that spend public funds or enjoy tax advantages should examine whether having providers of their services in positions of authority over the governance of the same agency or institution is in the best interest of that agency or institution or the services that are provided.

D. Where providers now sit on boards such as on Hospital Boards of Trustees, Blue Cross and Blue Shield Boards, Regional

Medical Programs, Boards of Health and various planning councils, they often are in "conflict of interest" positions and, in effect, decide what health services to purchase from themselves. When this occurs, these providers should be replaced by consumers or by professionals who cannot provide services under the authority of the agency they help control.

E. Where providers are not in such "conflict of interest" roles, they may play an essential part in the decision-making process. But those who derive income and profit from a specific system of health care should not be in a position to be advocate-judge-and-jury of those services.*

These consumer-oriented recommendations are discussed by two reviewers as they consider technology and health care systems in the 1980s. What is more important is the fact that one author is concerned with consumer-defined goals[62] and the other with consumer expectations of technology.[63] Coming as these articles do in a volume filled with professionals talking about the same futuristic picture of technology makes them all the more important. This is one of the few instances where any consideration has been given to the consumer viewpoint regarding medical technology.

Another set of recommendations, with more of a leaning toward the professional provider stance, have been proposed by the federal Office of Technology Assessment.[64] These are spelled out briefly below:

Policy alternatives presented in this report are grouped into five sections. The first section discusses alternatives to current Federal assessment activities both in terms of their expansion or change and the extent of that potential expansion. The other four sections correspond to the four steps in the assessment model. Each of these sections presents a number of options concerning the organizational location of the four functions of assessment. Following is a brief outline of these options:

Section One: Congressional Alternatives

Alternative A-1: Changes or expansions in the development of information concerning the safety and efficacy of

**Heal Yourself, Report of the Citizen's Board of Inquiry into Health Services for Americans,* American Public Health Association, 1971, p. 28.

medical technologies could occur solely in the private sector. This alternative would give the Federal Government the role of stimulating the private sector and monitoring its activities.

A-2: The Federal Government could expand its activities relating to the development of information on efficacy and safety of medical technologies. In this alternative, legislation could mandate the performance of certain activities.

A-3: Some combination of Alternatives A-1 and A-2 could be pursued.

Section Two: Identifying Technologies That Need Assessment

Alternative B-1. A new commission
B-2. Institute of Medicine
B-3. National Institutes of Health
B-4. Agencies involved in technology development
B-5. Food and Drug Administration
B-6. A new Federal office or agency, or the Office of Health Technology

Section Three: Requiring, Stimulating, Conducting, or Funding Studies

Alternative C-1. National Institutes of Health
C-2. Other Federal agencies
C-3. Food and Drug Administration
C-4. A new Federal office or agency, or the Office of Health Technology

Section Four: Synthesizing Information

Alternative D-1. A new commission
D-2. Institute of Medicine
D-3. National Institutes of Health
D-4. Agencies involved in technology development
D-5. Food and Drug Administration
D-6. Office of Health Practice Assessment
D-7. A new Federal office or agency, or the Office of Health Technology

Section Five: Disseminating Information

Alternative E-1. National Institutes of Health
E-2. Other Federal agencies

E-3. A new Federal office or agency, or the Office of Health Technology
E-4. A new office in the Department of Health, Education, and Welfare

The task of identifying technologies that need assessment could be assigned to any of the agencies listed in B-1 through B-6. Essentially, the alternatives are concerned with the advantages and disadvantages of each agency in achieving its function.

Any of the alternative agencies in section three could expand the support for the testing of technologies regarding safety and efficacy. C-1 and C-3 have had considerable experience in this area.

The alternative agencies in section four could synthesize the information with a critical eye toward gaps and needs. Data must be open to the public and other interested parties. This agency should also have professional and public visibility.

Any of the agencies in section five could identify those parties needing the information and develop, improve, or expand communications channels to appropriate parties. Agencies should also evaluate the impact of the information and determine whether the needs for data are being met.

These Office of Technology Assessment recommendations do not spell out the role of the consumer in the organizational procedures. Perhaps a combination of the two groups of recommendations would make more sense to consumers. Roles for consumers would have to be specified within the newly created agencies or the existing agencies and assigned tasks as suggested in the various sections. This skeleton is professionally organized and assumes the dominance of the providers. Obviously, the OTA recommendations would require some tempering with a consumer viewpoint.

A net effect would be the integration of the consumer attitudes and participation into the workings of the governmental controlled framework outlined in the second group of recommendations. Furthermore, this type of organizational system would have to be translated into geographically determined patterns, perhaps akin to the 205 health service area designations.

To offset the profound tones of the consumer and professional recommendations, consumers can consider the space age decision-making powers conferred within the cybernated world of ultimate technologic health care.

Space Age Recommendations

Workings of the New Medical Order[65] establishes a system where more bits of data will be available in the total health care process with less error and greater range. This Postphysician Era will consist of the following:

Inputers who feed data to the computer such as Ph.D.s, researchers, and programmers
Computers to mechanically handle the workload
Outputers who will be concerned with the delivery of services such as nurses, social workers, and allied health personnel
Patients who supply the warm bodies when in need of services
Synthesizers such as planners, evaluators, and administrators
Leaders who will be the creative synthetic executives of the system

Schools of Humanistic Medicine would teach philosophy, ethics, psychology, human communication, sociology, and other courses to the students. Students will take classes together and come from the ranks of the inputers, outputers, synthesizers, and leaders. However, despite the dependence upon the experts, there must be a constant dialogue with the public. Obviously, there is an assumption that the experts are all altruistic and have the public good as their overall imperative. In the best of all worlds, this may be so. Maybe consumers have something to look foward to in the future.

SUMMARY AND CONCLUSION

Technology is an accepted part of American culture and is growing more so each day. This is reflected in the development of the health care delivery system. In the past, there would be little questioning of the introduction of new medical technologies into the health care system. Everybody accepted the new drugs, devices, and techniques. This was especially so in as the third party payers picked up the tab for most of the expenses. However, the soaring inflationary spiral finally caught up with the health care system and "cost containment" became the overrriding catchword. Technology started to sprout the villain's appearance.

Included in legislative efforts to control costs were mandates for consumers to be majority participants in situations where decisions about medical care technology were to be made. Obviously, consumers had to learn the language of technology in rudimentary fashion. Furthermore, consumers had to learn to meet with health care providers on an equal footing and to demand explanations in plain and simple language.

Cherished values and attitudes held by both providers and consumers influence their reactions to technological advances and their reactions to each other in the newly created decision-making situations. Consumer values include a strange mix of faith in technology to solve all ailments along with a growing uneasiness as mass media recounted more and more failures relative to radiation dangers, toxic chemical dumpings, and occupational hazards. Provider values included a well-honed desire to use the biggest and the best that technology had to offer. This attitude was nourished during their professional education and in their clinical internships. Furthermore, the decision-making power of the provider was held as a sacrosanct right because of their training and experience. What was the consumer going to contribute to the evaluation of medical care technology? Into this seemingly adversary stance, the consumer must be strong enough to adopt a critical position and represent the values of the individual patient as well as the public good view of the total community.

Organizationally, the evolution of the medical care system, the specific aspects of technology development, and the accomplishments of technology, all influence the structure of the health care delivery system. Since the medical care establishment has been in the forefront of the leadership, the organizational efforts have moved toward high technology utilization. Consumers must learn about techniques used to make decisions about organizational structures and secure aid from staff in pursuing that route of assessment. Interestingly enough, many common medical procedures such as appendectomies and tonsillectomies, have been integrated into health care organizational patterns without the critical approach. Now, these procedures are being questioned as to their safety and efficacy.

The costs of medical technology are a critical topic for decision makers. Consumers must be alert to the fact that it is extremely difficult to place a price tag on lives saved, diseases prevented, disability lessened, or the discomfort of pain. Studies exist that support both the savings accumulated by the use of technology and increase in expenditures due to technology. Consumers will have to press for rationales for the cost figures and search for a direct relationship between the process of care and the outcome to the patient.

Roles for consumers in the medical technology process have to be developed as consumers become more active in the process. Consumers have not had that much experience in the decision-making role. Of major importance is the need to educate the consumer to participate on an equal footing. This may involve establishing consumer information networks and other data-generating devices. Obviously, consumers will need inner strength to speak up at meetings and to hold their position until their questions are answered.

Recommendations affect both the providers and consumers. Efforts can be made to shore up deficits in the established organizational system and to create the atmosphere in which consumers can thrive. In any event, the ultimate goal should seek the active cooperation of providers and consumers in working toward the most desirable public good for the total community.

As a concluding exhibit, Table 1-3 compares the tech-

Table 1–3 A Historical Technological Parable ?

X-ray	*CAT scan*
Discovery	
"Somatic illumination by Electricity . . . Two electrical discoverers report about simultaneously new medical and surgical uses for an extremely powerful light . . . . Professor Roentgen, the well-known professor of Wurzburg University . . . is said to have photographed the bones of the hand, all the soft parts being invisible . . . ." February 1, 1896, Journal of the American Medical Association[1]	"A new and fundamentally different x-ray method is described . . . . Modern electronic and computer technology have been allied to x-ray detection and measurement . . . in such a way that remarkable tissue differentiation becomes possible." December 1973, British Journal of Radiology[2]
"The further fact, that in a general way only the density of the medium penetrated seems to affect them ("the x-rays") . . . hints at future valuable physiologic revelations as well as diagnostic aids. It is only a hint however, and whether it is to be ever realized to any extent is perhaps open to serious question." February 15, 1896, Journal of the American Medical Association[3]	"Computerized axial tomography (CAT) has proved to be a revolutionary and reliable method of detecting intracranial pathology . . . limitations of space and specimen study in the EMI scanner make it difficult to predict the future utility of total body scanning." June, 1975, American Journal of Roentgenology[4]
". . . that we have a force, for that is what it may be called, that will act . . . through flesh, cartilage, skin and other tissues of the animal body, is enough to be fertile of practical suggestions to any thinking physician or surgeon." February 15, 1896, Journal of the American Medical Association[3]	

Table 1-3 Continued

X-ray	*CAT scan*
Utilization	
"In late February, 1896 . . . begged me to make an x-ray photograph of his hand and thus enable Dr. Bull to locate the numerous shot and extract them. The first attempts were unsuccessful because the patient was too weak and too nervous to stand a photographic exposure of nearly an hour. My good friend, Thomas Edison, had sent me several most excellent fluorescent screens . . . . I decided to try a combination of Edison's fluorescent screens and the photographic plate. The fluorescent screen was placed on the photographic plate and the patient's hand was placed upon the screen . . . . The combination succeeded, even better than I had expected. A beautiful photograph was obtained with the exposure of a fe seconds. The photographic plate showed the numerous shot as if they had been drawn with pen and ink . . . ."[9]	"Although the newness of CAT and our relative inexperience with a large number of cases make us hesitant at present to draw any firm conclusions with respect to this procedure, this early survey has encouraged us." January 1974, Mayo Clinic Proceedings[5]
"Many uses are suggested to which this ray can be put, and the newspapers are full of experimental researches in this country and abroad. We find that many universities in the East, as well as our own, are making experiments . . . Out of all this work must proceed some good." February 29, 1896, Journal of the American Medical Association[6]	"After considerable experimentation with animals, Hounsfield and J. E. A. Ambrose were ready for their first patient in October, 1971. The result exceeded their expectations, in that they demonstrated the cerebral ventricles clearly and also showed a well demarcated tumour in the left frontal lobe. The brain was no longer mute to x-rays." June, 1974, British Medical Journal[7]
"One of the most unexpected . . . but obviously one of the most useful applications of the x-ray is in the study of soft tissues which do not cast a sharp shadow as bones or calcium do." July 4, 1896, Medical Records, New York[16]	

Table 1–3 Continued

X-ray	*CAT scan*
Utilization (continued)	
"The surgeons of Vienna and Berlin believe that the Roentgen photograph is destined to render inestimable services to surgery . . . . Half an hour is the shortest exposure possible, and most require an hour." March 7, 1896, Journal of the American Medical Association[8]	"Computer assisted tomography appears to represent a major advance in neuroradiologic diagnosis and in the care of patients with neurologic disorders . . . . The major disadvantages of computer assisted tomography relate to its inherent characteristics such as the relative slowness of scanning and the limitation in viewing capability, both of which restrict the number of diagnostic procedures to 15 per day." January 1974, Mayo Clinic Proceedings[5]
Costs	
"Roentgen Photograph . . . . The electric apparatus required is so expensive, $100.00 and upward, that few surgeons can use it yet in their private practice." March 7, 1896, Journal of the American Medical Association[8]	"CAT fever has reached epidemic proportions and continues to spread among physicians, manufacturers, entrepreneurs and regulatory agencies. A cursory review of any radiologic or neuroscience journal attests to the virulence of this new disease. Within the United States alone, the costs of this epidemic are staggering . . . . The capital cost for just the computed tomographic units have been estimated, at today's prices, as 1.2 billion dollars over the next decade (Abramowitz K: Unpublished data)." April 22, 1976, New England Journal of Medicine[11]
	"Why, when the cost of medicine is under attack, does the profession and society indulge itself in such ultra-expensive new technology? The author believes it to be a unique conditioning of our times.

Table 1–3 Continued

X-ray	*CAT scan*
Costs (continued)	
	. . . thus, rather than wait the four weeks for a study on the outpatient list, the outpatient is admitted and obtains the study within a few days as an inpatient. The hospital has sweetened the $200+ scan with several days hospitalization at $150 per day. Good business, yes, but perhaps bad medicine."[14]
Honors	
"Honor for Professor Roentgen: The Prince Regent of Bavaria has conferred upon Professor Roentgen, of Wurzberg, the Knights Cross, one of the Bavarian orders . . ." March 21, 1896, British Medical Journal[12]	"Mr. G. N. Hounsfield and E. M. I. Ltd. were honored recently by receiving the MacRobert Award which is 'presented by the Council of Engineering Institutions on behalf of the MacRobert Trust for successful technological innovation which contributed or will contribute to national prestige and prosperity of the United Kingdom'." December 1973, British Journal of Radiology[13]
Side effects	
"The Roentgen Ray as a Moral Agent . . . the case of a young woman who applied for an operation on account of pain in her arm, as she was convinced that there was some abnormal condition of the bone. The surgeon . . . by taking a photograph of the arm, proved to her that it was perfect. Once convinced of this, the patient left entirely cured." April 25, 1896, Journal of the American Medical Association[15]	". . . Baker has cited a clear drop in the number of radionuclide brain scans, echoencephalograms and pneumoencephalograms as a result of the introduction of computed tomography. But Baker's analysis did not address the critical issues of costs, sensitivity or specificity of these procedures, nor did it recognize the distinction between need and demand . . . the physicians control demand and demand cannot be adduced as the final and only index of need." April 22, 1976, New England Journal of Medicine[11]

Table 1–3 Continued

X-ray	*CAT scan*
Critical notes	
"Once reasonable critique prevailed over the initial flurry of unreasonable expectations from Wilhelm Roentgen's discovery in 1895, practical experiments with the new rays were initiated in numerous scientific communities. It then seemed that the art of medicine, and especially of surgery, would be denied the anticipated gains in diagnosis and that our far reaching hopes were all to no avail. Were not the initial exposure times so long, several hours being required for larger parts of the body, that it seemed impossible to force the living human body and its extremities to remain immobile sufficiently long.... In recent times we have not exceeded five minutes for any exposure. On the average, one-half to one minute are sufficient for the exposure of a child's pelvis or comparably sized anatomic part. Similarly, very short ("momentary") exposures are adequate to make sharp, immaculate pictures of the hand and forearm."[10]	"Granted that this new technique can give sensational images and granted that it can, in specific cases, provide vital and perhaps lifesaving information, its relation to other well established and less costly neuroradiologic procedures is as yet undefined and fundamental questions remain to be answered about the relative cost effectiveness of the new computed tomographic scanners. The history of technologic advances in medicine is replete with examples of radiologic and surgical techniques that have ultimately been judged nonefficacious . . . doubtless, there is a subset of patients who will benefit from any of these generally unwarranted procedures . . . ." April 22, 1976, New England Journal of Medicine[11]
Future	
"Physicians from time immemorial have ever had a keen desire to explore the interior of the animal body. Hence arose dissection, and later on vivisection, and still later on the revelations of the microscope. But none of these methods fully satisfied the wish to know what is actually taking place within the animal organism during life . . . . No wonder then that the x-ray with its marvelous revelations of the hitherto unseen has excited universal interest." July 4, 1896, Medical Records, New York[16]	

Table 1–3 Continued

X-ray	*CAT scan*
Future	
"Gentlemen: I am convinced that I have not been able to tell you much that was not already known to you, and that some of you could show pictures made with perhaps even shorter exposures . . . . As we review the progress that has been made since we last met a year ago, we are surely entitled to the opinion that we have not yet arrived at the goal of the attainable. With concerted and continued effort, surely we are permitted the hope to illuminate other so far obscured organs and pathologic lesions of the human body with the help of the new light ray." April 22, 1897, Dr. Hermann Kummell, Berlin[10]	*DEPARTMENT OF HEALTH, EDUCATION, AND WELFARE* *Health Resources Administration* *[42 CFR Part 121]* *NATIONAL GUIDELINES FOR HEALTH PLANNING* *Advance Notice of Proposed Rulemaking* AGENCY: Public Health Service, HEW. ACTION: Notice of Proposed Rulemaking. X. COMPUTED TOMOGRAPHIC SCANNERS GUIDELINES [2] "A Policy Statement: Computed Tomoner (head and body) should operate at a minimum of 2,500 patient procedures per year. B. There should be no CT scanners approved unless each existing or approved CT scanner in the service area is performing at a rate greater than 4,000 patient procedures per year. C. Charges for existing or proposed CT scanner are to be calculated on the basis of 2,500, the projected or actual number of patient procedures per year, whichever is greater. D. There should be no new computed tomographic (CT) scanners approved unless the owners or operators of the proposed equipment will set in place, with operation of the equipment, a data collection system. DISCUSSION Because CT scanners are expensive to purchase, to maintain, and to staff, every effort must be made to contain costs while providing an acceptable level of service. Full and appropriate utilization of existing units will pre-

Table 1–3 Continued

X-ray	*CAT scan*
	vent needless duplication and limit unnecessary increases in health care costs. Estimates of full utilization of CT scanners range from 1,800 to 4,000 patient procedures per year. Surveys of actual usage show a slightly wider range. The Institute of Medicine, provider organizations, and specialists who have carefully reviewed these data and analyzed the capabilities of various commercially available units have recommended that 2,500 patient procedures per year be considered as the minimal acceptable number for adequate utilization. Prior to opening more than one CT Scanner in a service area, existing clinical units should be operating at a maximum level. A summary of the data collected on CT scanners should be submitted by the owners or operators to the appropriate HSA, to enable the Agency to adequately plan distribution and use of CT scanners in the area. The data to be collected should include the following:[2] Presenting signs and symptoms of CT examinations. Demographic characteristics of recipients of CT examinations. Rate of positive diagnoses of different disease conditions by CT. Place of CT examinations in sequence with other diagnostic procedures. Sensitivity and specificity of CT examinations performed in different parts of the body. Federal Register September 23, 1977

Table 1–3 Continued

REFERENCES

1. Unidentified writer. Miscellany section. *Journal of the American Medical Association*, 1896, *26*, 244–245.
2. Ambrose J. Computerized transverse axial scanning (tomography): Part 2. Clinical application. *British Journal of Radiology*, 1973, *46*, 1023–1047.
3. Unidentified writer. Miscellany section. *Journal of the American Medical Association*, 1896, *26*, 336.
4. Alfidi RJ, MacIntyre WJ, Meaney TF, et al. Experimental studies to determine application of CAT scanning to the human body. *American Journal of Roentgenology*, 1975, *124*, 199–207.
5. Baker HL, Campbell JK, Houser DW, et al. Computer assisted tomography of the head. *Mayo Clinic Proceedings*, 1974, *49*, 17–27.
6. Burry J. A preliminary report on the Roentgen or x-rays. *Journal of the American Medical Association*, 1896, *26*, 402–404.
7. Unidentified editorial writer. Computer assisted tomography. *British Medical Journal*, 1974, *2*, 623–624.
8. Unidentified writer. Miscellany section. *Journal of the American Medical Association*, 1896, *26*, 491.
9. Pupin M. *From immigrant to inventor*. New York: Charles Scribner's Sons, 1930.
10. Kümmel H. The significance of Roentgen's ray for surgery. V. Langenbeck's *Arch Clin Chir*, 1897, *55*, 194–210 (Author's translation).
11. Shapiro SH, Wyman SM. CAT fever. *New England Journal of Medicine*, 1976, *294*, 954–956.
12. Unidentified writer. Special correspondence. *British Medical Journal*, 1896, *1* (1896), 756.
13. Unidentified editorial. *British Journal of Radiology*, 1973, *46*, 1015.
14. Freedman GS. Computerized tomography—development and impact on nuclear medicine and other health services and medical economics. In: Bennington JL, Boer GB, Louvau GE, Westlake GE: Management and Cost Control Techniques for the Clinical Laboratory. University Park Press, Baltimore, in press, pp. 135–152.
15. Unidentified writer. *Journal of the American Medical Association*, 1896, *26*, 843–844.
16. Morton WJ. The "x"-ray and some of its applications in medicine—demonstrations of apparatus at work and exhibition of stereopticon views. *Medical Records* (New York) *50*, 9–11.

Source: R. L. Schapiro, "Opinions of an Editor," *Journal of Computed Axial Tomography*, 1977 (1):1–7.

nologic developments of the x-ray and the CAT scanner. Actual quotes illustrate opinions about the discovery, the utilization, the costs, the honors awarded, the side effects, the critical comments, and the future of each advance. Readers can look between the lines and come to their own conclusions as to the moral of the technological parable.

REFERENCES

1. Rettig, R. A. *Health care technology: Lessons learned from the end-stage renal disease experience.* Santa Monica, Ca.: *The Rand Paper Series,* 1976, p. 8.

2. Office of Technology Assessment. *Assessing the efficacy and safety of medical technologies.* Washington, D.C.: U.S. Gov't. Printing Office, 1978, p. 107.
3. Rettig, *Health care technology* p. 1.
4. Office of Technology Assessment. *Development of medical technology.* Washington, D.C.: U.S. Govt. Printing Office, 1976, p. 45.
5. Green, H. Limitations on implementation of technology assessment. *Atomic Energy Law Journal,* 1972, *14,* 61.
6. Office of Technology Assessment, *Assessing medical technologies,* p. 14.
7. Abernathy, W. J., Sheldon, A., & Prahalad, C. K. *The management of health care.* Cambridge, Ma.: Ballinger, 1974, p. 267.
8. Ibid., p. 7.
9. Steiger, W. A. Medical science and things. *Health and Human Behavior,* 1964, *4(1),* 39.
10. Beall, A. C., Jr. Heart valve prostheses: Who protects our patients, and from what? *Medical Instrumentation,* 1977, *11,* 72.
11. Carlson, R. J. Business as usual? in R. H. Egdahl & P. M. Gertman (Eds.). *Technology and the quality of health care.* Germantown, Md.: Aspen Systems Corp., 1978, p. 51.
12. Ibid., p. 50.
13. National Academy of Sciences. *How safe is safe. The design of policy on drugs and food additives.* Washington, D. C., 1974. Advisory Committee on Industrial Innovations.
14. USDHEW. *Forward Plan for Health, 1977–1981.* Washington, D.C.: U.S. Gov't. Printing Office, 1975. p. 93.
15. Industrial Innovation Coordinating Committee. *Review and recommendations of policy alternatives of the public interest advisory subcommittee: Draft Report.* Washington, D.C.: Advisory Committee on Industrial Innovations 1978.
16. Cambridge Research Institute. *Trends affecting the U.S. health care system.* Cambridge, Ma.: DHEW Pub. No. HRA 76-14503 Cambridge, Ma.: 1975, p. I–32.
17. Abernathy et al. *The management of health care,* p. 100.
18. Tancredi, L. R., & Barsky, A. J. Technology and health care decision making—conceptualizing the process for societal informed consent. *Medical Care,* 1974, *12,* 845.
19. Carlson, *Business as usual?* p. 46.
20. Office of Technology Assessment, *Assessing medical technologies,* p. 108.

21. Rettig, R. A. End-stage renal disease and the "cost" of medical technology. Santa Monica, Ca.: *The Rand Paper Series.* 1977, p.11.
22. Carlson, *Business as usual?* p. 47.
23. Nelson, R. Issues and suggestions for the study of industrial organization in a regime of rapid technical change, in V. R. Fuchs (Ed.). *Policy issues and research opportunities in industrial organization.* New York, National Bureau of Economic Research, 1972.
24. Lewin and Associates, Inc. *Evaluation of the efficiency and effectiveness of the section 1122 review process.* Washington, D.C. 1975.
25. Abt Associates, Inc. *Incentives and decisions underlying hospitals' adoption and utilization of major capital equipment: executive summary.* Cambridge, Ma. September, 1975.
26. Cathcart, R. Doing more with less—gracefully. *Trustee,* 1978, *31,* 17.
27. Parker, B. R. Quantitative decision techniques for the health public sector policy-maker: An analysis and classification of resources. *Journal of Health Politics, Policy and Law,* 1978, *3(3),* 388.
28. Kosowsky, D. in Egdahl and Gertman, *Technology and the quality of health care,* p. 272.
29. Barnard, C., & Pepper, C. B. *One life.* New York: Macmillan, 1969, p. 311.
30. Maxmen, J. S., Goodbye Dr. Welby. *Social Policy 1973, 3(4&5)*, 97.
31. Ibid., Roszak, T., p. 106.
32. Computer use may raise risk of malpractice. *Medical Tribune,* 1969.
33. Schoolman, H. M., & Bernstein, L. M. Computer use in diagnosis, prognosis, and therapy. *Science,* 1978, *200* 926.
34. Office of Technology Assessment, *Development of medical technology,* 1978 pp. 26–55.
35. Brown, J. H. U., & Dickson III, J. F. Instrumentation and the delivery of health services. *Science,* 1969, *166,* 334.
36. Denison, E., quoted in Hanley, J. W. The can-do spirit. *Newsweek,* January 8, 1979 p. 7.
37. Office of Technology Assessment, *Development of medical technology,* 1978, p. 15.
38. McPherson, K., & Fox, M. S. Treatment of breast cancer, in J. P. Bunker et al. (Eds.) *Costs, risks, and benefits of surgery.* New York: Oxford University Press, 1977.
39. Gordis, L. Naggan, L., & Tonascia, J. Pitfalls in evaluating the impact

of coronary care units on mortality from myocardial infarctions. *John Hopkins Medical Journal,* 1977, *141,* 287.

40. Mather, H. G., Pearson, N. G., Read, K. L., Q., et al. Acute myocardial infarction: Home and hospital treatment. *British Medical Journal,* 1971, *3,* 334.
41. Maugh, T. H. Diabetes therapy: Can new techniques halt complications? *Science, 1975, 190,* 1281.
42. Chalmers, T. C. Settling the UGDP controversy. *Journal of the American Medical Association,* 1975, *231,* 624.
43. Barach, A. L. The indiscriminate use of IPPB. *Journal of the American Medical Association,* 1967, *231,* 1141.
44. Baroon, S., & Wolfe, H. *Measuring the effectiveness of medical decisions.* Springfield, Ill.: Charles C Thomas, 1972.
45. Lampert, R. P., Robinson, D. S., Soyka, L. F. A critical look at oral decongestants. *Pediatrics,* 1975, *55,* 550.
46. Moskowitz, M., Milbrath, J., Gartside, P., et. al. Lack of efficacy of thermography as a screening tool for minimal and stage I breast cancer. *New England Journal of Medicine,* 1976, *295,* 249.
47. Waters, W. E. Controlled clinical trial of ergotamine tartrate. *British Medical Journal* 1970, *2* (5705), 325–327.
48. Seeff, L. B., Zimmerman, H. J., Wright, E. C., et. al. A randomized double blind controlled trial of the efficacy of immune serum globulin for the prevention of post-transfusion hepatitis. *Gastroenterology,* 1977, *72,* 111.
49. Griner, P. F. Treatment of acute pulmonary edema: Conventional or intensive care? *Annals of Internal Medicine,* 1972, *77,* 501.
50. Cambridge Research Institute, *Trends,* p. 1–38.
51. Spiegel, A. D., & Backhaut, B. *Factors affecting the quality of health care.* Springfield, Va.: National Technical Information Service, 1977.
52. Spiegel, A. D. *Factors affecting the acceptability of health care.* Springfield, Va.: National Technical Information Service, 1978.
53. Gaus, C. in Egdahl and Gertman, *Technology and the quality of health care* p. 278.
54. Dubos, R. *The mirage of health.* New York: Harper & Row, 1971, p. 130.
55. Somers, A. R. Health care and the political system: The sorcerer's apprentice revisited, in M. Collen (Ed.). *Technology and health care*

systems in the 1980s. Washington, D.C.: National Center for Health Services Research, 1973, p. 42.

56. Ibid., Anderson, O. W., Medical technology and the political system, p. 36.
57. Caceres, C., in Egdahl and Gertman, *Technology and the quality of health care,* p. 271.
58. Rettig, *Health care technology,* p. 25.
59. Crawford, R. You are dangerous to your health—The ideology and politics of victim blaming. *International Journal of Health Services, 1977, 7,* 663.
60. Doong, J. *Consumer participation in health planning: An annotated bibliography.* DHEW Pub. No. (HRA) 77-14551. Washington, D.C.: U.S. Gov't Printing Office, 1976.
61. American Public Health Association. *Heal yourself. Report of the Citizen's Board of Inquiry into Health Services for Americans,* Washington, D.C. 1971. p. 28.
62. Breslow L. Consumer defined goals for the health care systems of the 1980s, in M. Collen (Ed.). *Technology and health care systems in the 1980s.* Washington, D.C.: National Center for Health Services Research, 1973.
63. Ibid., Spencer, W. A. Consumer expectations of technology, p. 125.
64. Office of Technology Assessment, *Assessing medical technologies,* 1978 pp. 97–103.
65. Maxmen, J. S., *Goodbye Dr. Welby,* p. 102.

Part I

MEDICAL TECHNOLOGY AND THE HEALTH CARE CONSUMER

Anticipating the idea that many of the people who would attend the conference series would be coming to more than one of the four sessions, this opening conference was designed to set a foundation upon which the following conferences would build. Basic themes were discussed, including a debate concerning the value of medical technology, the argument over the expertise of the consumer as compared to the professional, and an overview of medical technology. Afternoon workshops also concentrated on basics by exploring consumer evaluation of medical technology, patients' rights and informed consent, medical statistics, and the consumers' role in health planning decisions.

All of these issues had been raised in meetings of the Project Advisory Committee. In the discussions the point was made repeatedly that the average consumer serving on health-related governing boards and committees was not as well prepared as the professional to render decisions. Lack of information was a major impediment to consumer effectiveness. In addition, the consumer had to gain the confidence to speak up at meetings and to play an assertive role in the decision-making process. Medical mystique, the inate ability of physicians to assume God-like mantles, that age old problem, was considered by the Project Advisory Committee to be a decisive factor in inducing consumer reticence at governing board meetings.

Workshops in the afternoon were planned to allow the audience to ask questions about topics usually reserved for health care professionals: the evaluation of health care, the rights of patients, the confusion of statistical numbers, and the secretive decisions in executive offices. It was reasoned that the audience would be able to explore these areas in depth within smaller groups with a fruitful exchange ensuing. From the evaluation questionnaires, it appeared that the participants felt that this aim was achieved.

In his opening address, Peter Rogatz presented a wide ranging overview of the impact of technology on medical care. At the beginning of the talk several questions were posed such as, "Shall we do everything possible to extend every patient's life regardless of cost?" and "Shall we do everything regardless of whether there is an expectation of restoring the patient to a useful social role?" Obviously, these questions have expansive ramifications regarding the impact of medical technology. Issues like these merely pinpoint a portion of the complexities that the consumers and providers face regarding concerns about the use of technology in health care.

Following a recounting of the historical relationship of technology to health care and noting the changing values along the way, Rogatz cited the advantages and disadvantages resulting from the use of technology in medicine. While a major advantage appeared to be the great reduction in death and sickness, the point was also made that mortality and morbidity rates were falling prior to the introduction of various medical technologies. Increased life expectancy has been attributed to the improvements in environmental sanitation, nutrition, and housing rather than medical advances. There are other nonmedical advantages, however, which technology brings to health care such as the ability to transmit information and to conduct efficient screening programs. Disadvantages include the urge to exercise the technologic imperative, a concomitant depersonalization along with advanced technology and actual illness that can be traced to the introduction of medical technology. Rogatz discussed the examples of problems arising from transfusions, mammography, fetal monitoring, and human and/or mechanical errors associated with laboratory testing. Some ethical dilemmas were also cited regarding technology and health care such as the issue of abortions, life-sustaining regimens, use of artificial organs, genetic research, and, even, cloning.

In conclusion, Rogatz spoke about the mixed blessings of medical technology and the concept of "overdoctoring." Technology has to be considered in relation to the expectations of specific social benefits for the whole society as well as those for a particular individual.

As the first speaker in a debate on the pros and cons of a better life through the use of medical technology, Stewart identified the issues for debate. He pointed out that distinctions should be made between disagreements about facts and disagreements about values. Costs and benefits are also affected by this separation of facts and values and must be regarded in the total discussion. Stewart noted that evidence could be mustered to support either side of the argument that medical technology is effective or that medical technology is ineffective. Is it really a direct result of the application of medical technology or are there other variables such as socioeconomic factors that produce the desired reductions in death and illness? While commenting that he was not dead set against technology, Stewart stated that hard choices had to be made between socially desirable alternatives. An example was given of the choice of expending funds for improved maternal care services or for more neonatal and infant care services. Is there any reasonable way to make such a choice? Related to this problem is the assessment of medical technology. Efficacy and safety are the two issues raised most often, followed closely by cost factors. Stewart concluded that consumers who are involved in these difficult decisions should be well informed regardless of whether they are pro- or antitechnology.

Del Guercio commented that the antitechnology movement in the United States is causing this nation to lose its once impressive lead in medicine. CAT scanners and artificial hip joints, two newer innovations, were both developed in Britain. Furthermore, Del Guercio stated that technology should not be made the scapegoat for the enormous increases in health care costs; 55 percent can be attributed to inflation and less than 4 percent to an increase in the use of technology. A plea was made to reduce health care costs through the application of cost-lowering technology itself such as ambulatory surgical centers, medical information systems, and the effective evaluation of preoperative risk. Citing the supportive comments of Nobel prize winners, Del Guercio called for the resuscitation of technical innovation. Technologic entrepreneurs were called an endangered species who are overregulated and undersupported. He summed up by saying that medical technology is our only hope for containing costs and improving the quality of care.

Levin and Light addressed themselves to the question of who is the expert in health care decision making. Levin presented the consumer view while Light gave the health professional's side. Noting the firm placement of consumerism in the medical care field, Levin also pointed out the reluctance of consumers to participate in the decision-making process on an equal footing. He attributed this to the "mystique" of medicine, science, and technology. Levin proceeded to distinguish between experts and consumers with particular attention to disagreements among experts. If experts disagree, then consumers must learn to heed their own counsel. Consumers must listen to all sides and, according to Levin, come to a fair decision. Gaining access to understandable information, however, presents consumers with a substantial problem. Professionals tend to sit on data and to write material using their own exotic jargon. Yet, Levin argued that consumers must overcome their timidity and pose critical questions to professionals and make them explain things in simple language. Levin commented, "Properly, the role of the professional-specialist is that of advisor to the consumer-generalist." Government should assist the consumer in achieving that role by ensuring the availability of information and by covering all sides of the issue. He concluded by answering the title question, "I would answer that the expert is the consumer-generalist in whom ultimate power should be vested."

Taking the provider side, Light disclaimed that there is an inherent adversary relationship between the health care provider and the health care consumer. He stated that the decision-making responsibility on the use of technology clearly rests with the consumer, except in cases of life and death emergencies. Several examples of the impact of medical technology were discussed including well publicized stories about a Bowery bum who refused to have his gangrenous leg amputated, the decisions regarding Jehovah's Witnesses, and health care decisions about the use of heroic life-saving measures and regarding "pulling the plug" on comatose patients who have no hope of recovery. Light concluded that he believed that the medical profession has been unfairly maligned in the area of patient's rights and in their respect for those rights. He did note, however, that physicians should be more sensitive to the dependent status of the individual who is ill and to that person's willingness to abrogate his or her decision-making responsibility. This sensitivity on the medical profession's part, Light feels, will enhance their status in the community, reduce their medicolegal difficulties and remove some of the burden from their shoulders.

In the afternoon workshops, basic issues were raised relative to the evaluation of health care, informed consent, statistics, and decision making.

In the workshop on what consumers should know about evaluating medical technology, a distinction was made between the concerns of consumers and providers. Consumer concerns were classified as primarily subjective while providers were concerned with objective analyses. Consumer participants at the workshop, however, pointed to the difference between consumers as patients and as members of health planning agencies. Although consumers wanted to familiarize themselves with criteria developed by providers, they also wished to develop their own standards. In fact, the consumer role was described by one panelist as "evaluating the evaluators."

"Patients' Rights and Informed Consent in a Technological Era" was the title of another workshop session. Panelists presented information on the aspects of patients' rights and informed consent from a legal and medical viewpoint. During the question-and-answer portion, the issue of "ghost surgery" was raised. Needs of medical teaching institutions entered the conversation relative to the rights of patients and the need to provide warm bodies for medical training purposes. This was followed by a heated discussion over how much physicians ought to tell their patients about the purposes and risks of medical procedures. Paternalism versus the individual's self-determination was seen as an underlying issue and was discussed at length.

Various statistical techniques were explained to the participants in the workshop on medical statistics and the health care consumer. Common terms such as length of stay, occupancy rate, incidence, and prevalence were illustrated, and their usage detailed. Problems with the use of data and the role of the consumer were discussed. Critical questions for consumers to keep in mind were also noted. Some questions were raised about using population based planning to make decisions for the future.

Another workshop focused on untangling the web of decision making in health planning and elucidating the role consumers do and/or should play in the process. While it was noted that the federal legislation mandates majority consumer participation, this will not come about without hard work. There were comparisons made between the degree of consumer power of the local Health Systems Agency (HSA) versus the state agency. A lack of communication between consumer members on HSAs and on State Health Coordinating Councils (SHCCs) was also discussed. Some discussion centered on the governmental obligations to educate and inform consumers and the formation of a consumer network was suggested.

Chapter 2

THE IMPACT OF TECHNOLOGY ON MEDICAL CARE: AN OVERVIEW

Peter Rogatz

Introduction

We have reached an extraordinary stage in the development of medical practice. As a result, we are confronted with questions of unprecedented difficulty. There was a time when a physician unhesitatingly would use every available means to diagnose and treat every patient's illness and to keep every patient alive as long as possible. No patient, no physician, and no outside observer questioned the appropriateness of this. Modern technology, however, has greatly complicated our view of the matter. Now we have diagnostic tools of astonishing complexity and ways of substituting machinery for body functions so as to prolong life for weeks, months, or years. Yet, far from solving problems, in many situations these new capabilities have produced cruel dilemmas for us.

Will every patient with symptoms receive maximum diagnostic study, regardless of cost? Will we do everything possible to extend every patient's life, regardless of cost? Will we do everything regardless of whether there is any expectation of restoring the patient to a useful social role or even of giving him or her a reasonable degree of physical and mental comfort? Will we insist upon continuing a patient's vital functions through the use of machinery even to the point where there is no certainty that the individual is alive by conventional criteria?

There is a characteristically American instinct—often described as "the technologic imperative"—which tells us that if something can be done, it must be done. Only recently have we begun to ask ourselves whether the unlimited application of medical technology involves costs greater than we can afford, or at least greater than the benefits that are likely to result. Each of us—even the professional provider of medical services—is fundamentally a health care consumer, and each of us must struggle with the very difficult questions posed by the explosive growth of medical technology.

To present an overview of the issues, the first section offers a brief historical perspective on the evolution of modern medical technology; the next two sections outline the salient advantages and disadvantages resulting from the use of technology; and the final section discusses some special dilemmas that demand special attention.

Historical Background

The first use of fire and the invention of stone tools, each dating back hundreds of thousands of years, are immeasurably significant technologic milestones in the history of the human race. Of much more recent vintage, the application of technology to the management of disease is more or less contemporaneous with the invention of the wheel a few thousand years ago. Some Egyptian mummies had teeth filled with gold, centainly a noteworthy technologic achievement.

The first hospitals may be discerned as far back as the 11th century B.C. Official houses were maintained in Egypt to which poor persons could go to receive treatment without charge by physicians paid by the government. Specialization, a facet of modern medical practice closely related to technology, was also known in ancient Egypt. According to Herodotus, "The art of medicine is thus divided among them; each physician applies himself to one disease only; some physicians are for the eye, others for the head, others for the teeth, others for the parts of the stomach and others for internal disorders."[1]

Thus, thousands of years ago, the beginnings of medicine, specialization, and technology were already in evidence. Ancient medicine, however, was intertwined with magical and religious practices. Throughout the millennia which followed those earliest beginnings the evolution of modern medicine has been marked by times of vital scientific endeavor interspersed with periods of regression to unsubstantiated dogma.

Hippocrates of Cos, teaching in the 4th and 5th centuries B.C., is widely credited with being the first to develop a scientific approach to medical practice. Several hundred years later, in the second century A.D., Galen of Pergamum became the next great medical innovator, discovering new facts about physiology, anatomy, disease processes, and the use of drugs.[2]

In the barbarian engulfment of the Roman empire, the knowledge of medicine accumulated by Hippocrates, Galen, and their pupils was largely lost to Europe. Fortunately, Avicenna, who studied, wrote, and taught under Arabian sponsorship in the 11th century, and Maimonides, the great Jewish scholar and philosopher of the 12th century, preserved and built upon the foundations laid by Hippocrates and Galen.

However, the Middle Ages in Europe were stagnant ones for medicine. Very little significant new knowledge was acquired. The few who applied scientific methods of inquiry (Roger Bacon outstanding among them) were virtually ignored, and dogma prevailed.

With the emergence of two giant figures—Paracelsus and Vesalius—the 16th century saw the beginnings of the modern experimental period. For the next 300 years, these men supplied the foundations upon which the scientific knowledge of medicine was laboriously constructed. Slowly, magic and mystery were replaced by experiment and knowledge. Understanding of human physiology was an essential step as exemplified by the discovery of the circulation of the blood by William Harvey in the early 17th century. Careful observation of diseases increased the ability to make diagnoses. On the other hand, lack of knowledge concerning underlying causation made effective treatment extremely difficult.

Throughout the 18th century, medicine and surgery were still seriously limited by insufficient understanding of disease processes, by lack of a method for relieving pain, and by inability to control infection. One extraordinary demonstration of medical technology was Edward Jenner's discovery (published in 1798) that inoculation with cowpox material could provide protection against smallpox.

A surge of major scientific developments emerged during the 19th century. If it were possible to identify the most critical milestones among the thousands of painstaking discoveries and innovations made during the 19th century, one would probably select the discovery of anesthesia by Dr. Crawford Long (1842) and Dr. William Morton (1846); the development of modern nursing practices by Florence Nightingale during the Crimean War (1854–1856); the bacteriologic discoveries of Louis Pasteur in the 1860s; and the development of antiseptic techniques by Joseph Lister during the same period. Countless others helped to pave the way with important discoveries of their own, but these pioneers opened the door finally and irrevocably to the development of modern medical and hospital practices. The era of technology in medicine was launched.

Around the turn of the 20th century, hospitals began to change from being largely caretakers of incurably ill patients to being places where specific treatment was provided. Specialities began to take shape and soon became an intrinsic part of the hospital structure. Throughout this century, hospitals underwent extraordinary growth and this expansion continues to this day.

Advantages Resulting from the Use of Technology

In the last quarter of the 20th century, we enjoy the benefits of scientific knowledge and technologic applications that would have been unimaginable only a few decades ago. It behooves us, however, to recognize that many important technologic contributions to our health preceded the development of the dramatic diagnostic and therapeutic tools that are the mainstay of the modern hospital.

Extraordinary declines in disease and death rates over the past two centuries are attributable much more to improvements in environmental sanitation, nutrition, and birth control than to medical advances.[3] Typhoid fever, scarlet fever, diarrhea, and enteritis—major killers in the late 19th century—succumbed to sanitary practices more than to medical treatment. Tuberculosis, whose conquest is sometimes attributed to the development of streptomycin and isoniazid in the mid-20th century, had lost much of its lethal potential long before the introduction of these drugs. We must recognize modern sanitary concepts as being among the great technologic advances of medical history, responsible for massive reductions in the occurrence of communicable diseases and related death rates.

Inoculation against smallpox and immunization against whooping cough, diptheria, and poliomyelitis also represent major triumphs. We usually take such preventive measures for granted although they actually represent outstanding examples of the application of technology in medicine. The current interest in medical technology, however, focuses mainly on diagnosis and treatment.

Doctors David Banta and Joshua Sanes defined medical technology as "the set of techniques, drugs, equipment, and procedures used by health care professionals in the delivery of clinical medical care to individuals."[4]

Radiology offers a prime example of medical technology at work. The era of modern diagnosis may be said to have begun with the discovery of x-rays by Dr. Wilhelm Roentgen in 1895. Years of patient investigation by many physicians and physicists gradually brought about the evolution of modern x-ray technology, producing pictures of extraordinary clarity and detail. (A tragic footnote and a significant commentary on modern technology as a "two-edged sword" are the history of the many martyrs who, before the dangers of radiology were properly understood, acquired a variety of cancers and x-ray burns in their efforts to improve the use of this new tool.)

A dramatic new chapter in the march of technology opened with the development of computed tomography (CT) scanning. Few medical tools have burst upon the world with such sudden impact as this device, which represents a combination of the marvels of x-ray diagnosis with computerization, which is probably familiar to every reader of weekly news magazines and Sunday newspaper supplements. There is no doubt that the new device provides diagnostic information with greater speed and safety that can be achieved through any other available techniques. There also is no question that, at an installation price of around half a million dollars, widespread application of this diagnostic tool will significantly impact on the costs of medical care.

If the impact on the effectiveness of diagnosis and treatment proves to be great enough, undoubtedly the cost will be worthwhile. At this time, there are significant differences of opinion as to whether the gains will justify the cost of installing CT scanners in numerous hospitals and free-standing facilities in almost every city across the country. One can find impassioned arguments on both sides of the question. It is tempting to believe that another few years experience with the manufacture and use of CT scanners will result in a reduction of cost and an improvement in the impact upon diagnosis and treatment. Whether such optimism will be borne out by events remains to be seen.

A word must be said here about screening techniques in modern health care. Of course, the appeal of these efforts lies in their potential for uncovering unsuspected illness. Yet, after an initial period of enthusiasm, there has been growing skepticism about mass screening for the following reasons:

> Yield of positive findings usually has been low relative to total cost.
>
> Our delivery system has failed to provide effective diagnostic follow-up and definitive treatment for patients with positive screening results.
>
> End results, in terms of mortality rates, are often not substantially better than the rates observed in the unscreened populations.

There are at least two areas, however, where screening, coupled with careful therapeutic follow-up, has been associated with reduced morbidity and mortality: Pap smears for early detection of cervical cancer and screening for early detection of hypertension. Although the results of such efforts are still the subject of debate, I think they are sufficiently promising to warrant optimism that effective screening approaches to other widely prevalent conditions eventually will be developed.

Technology has brought about a wide variety of new therapeutic approaches, some of which are dramatically successful and others disappointing; some gratifyingly inexpensive and others incredibly costly. Examples of highly effective yet relatively inexpensive treatment are the use of antibiotics and chemotherapy for the treatment of syphilis and tuberculosis and the use of hormone therapy for endocrine disorders. Dr. Lewis Thomas made the point that technology of this type, based upon "a genuine understanding of disease mechanisms . . . is relatively inexpensive, relatively simple and relatively easy to deliver."[5] By contrast, he refers to certain spectacular technologic approaches which do not strike at the underlying pathology or offer a fundamental cure, as "halfway technology." Thomas cites the examples of organ transplantation; kidney dialysis; treatment of cancer by surgery, irradiation, and chemotherapy; and the complex emergency teams and facilities developed to deal with myocardial infarction.

An essential point can be made: In the absence of a fundamental understanding of the underlying process, the best that medical science can accomplish against most diseases is to develop some type of complex technologic manipulation or gadgetry that modifies the anatomic and physiologic disturbances caused by disease. When fundamental knowledge of the underlying disease process is acquired, we are able to dispense with complex and costly machinery and substitute relatively simple and inexpensive therapy or, ideally, effective prevention. One need only contrast the complicated "iron lung" machine used in the 1940s to aid polio victims with the simplicity of today's vaccine to appreciate this point.

Another area that has profited from technology is the field of information. Our entire health care delivery system is impacted by the ability gained in recent years to process and transmit information at unprecedented speeds. Examples of this include the "hospital information systems" now in fairly widespread use; the more complex "medical information systems" still in a relatively rudimentary stage of development; the transmission of electrocardiography data by telephone with computer interpretation; and the use of closed circuit television to enable physicians to "see" and talk to patients in remote rural areas.

Sometimes one type of technology can be substituted for another, with benefit to the patient and reduced costs to the public as a whole. Thus, a study published recently by a team of investigators at Duke University[6] indicates that patients with uncomplicated heart attacks can be discharged safely from the hospital after seven days to convalesce at home, making use of telephone transmission of electrocardiography tracings to monitor their cardiac status. To the extent that this technique reduces the length of hospitalization, both the individual patient and society gain.

DISADVANTAGES RESULTING FROM THE USE OF TECHNOLOGY

Despite the advances, there are less happy consequences of technology, which fall into three major areas: the technologic imperative, depersonalization of medical care, and the occurrence of diseases and disorders that result from the use of technology.

The Technologic Imperative

A growing importance is attributed to the so-called technologic imperative, that seemingly irresistible impulse to acquire and use the newest, most complex, and most sophisticated technologic tools. In addition, the technologic imperative implies little concern with the proper evaluation of the tools, takes place with no proof that the tools are safe or even effective, and, in many cases, without regard for their cost. Walter McNerney[7] notes that many organizations have "an unspoken target of as much new technology as possible . . ." and tells of a proposal by "a large company to put a satellite over Southwest Indian Territory so that problems and treatment could be televised." He asks us to "pause to think of the investment in technical equipment and personnel this would involve and how absurd it would be in terms of population and simple primary care alternatives."

Although this is an extreme example, it is fair to say that the technologic imperative seems to have a firm grasp upon hospitals throughout the United States. Curiously, the phenomenon occurs more intensely in those settings where it is least needed: in urban areas where numerous hospitals exist. It would seem to be an unfortunate application of that cherished right of free enterprise: the right to compete with one's neighbor, or one's neighboring institutions.

Many factors contribute to this phenomenon. In some instances, it is the ego of a trustee who wants to boast that it was his or her gift that made it possible for the hospital to acquire an expensive new gadget. Sometimes it is the natural ambition of a hospital executive to see his/her institution grow to become "as good as" the other hospital in town. (It is unfortunate that "good" is so commonly equated with "large and complex.") In some cases it is the urge felt by a physician or group of physicians for their hospital to have the full range of diagnostic and therapeutic tools. This increases the variety and complexity of services they can offer and improves their reputations among both colleagues and patients.

Because of donations and because of the long-standing practice of third-party payers to reimburse without question for new equipment, hospitals have been able to command almost at will the capital resources needed to acquire new technologic tools. A belated recognition of the costly consequences of the technologic imperative can be seen in the passage of P.L. 93–641 (The National Health Planning and Resources Development Act of 1974) and in development of a more critical approach to reimbursement by many third-party payers. P.L. 93–641 mandated priorities to contain costs while maintaining the quality of health care.

Such constraints, however, are directed primarily at capital formation. There has been relatively little effective control over the use of these costly tools once they have been acquired. In the face of extensive health insurance, every hospital bed and every piece of equipment represents an invitation to overuse and abuse. Open heart surgery—an obvious but very important example of this problem—is not only an extremely costly service for a hospital to provide, but also one which involves unnecessary hazards if it is not performed in reasonably high volume. Skills needed for doing such surgery with minimum risk cannot be acquired and maintained if the team does not work frequently. Nevertheless, the majority of open-heart surgery units are functioning at levels well below the 200 cases per year established as a minimum standard by the Department of Health, Education and Welfare. Furthermore, Karen Davis,

Deputy Assistant Secretary for Health Planning and Evaluation, has reported that 80 percent of the hospitals where cardiac surgery currently is performed are not adequately staffed for this purpose.[8]

Another pertinent example is the CT scanners. It is estimated that the number of scanners currently in place or on order in the United States is about 1000. On a per capita basis, this is approximately ten times the number of machines in Great Britain, where the technology originated. Our scanner capacity in this country soon will be enough to provide 500 brain scans for every 1000 patients who consult physicians each year because of headache.[9] However, we should not abandon CT scanning as a technique for neurologic diagnosis. Rather, consideration should be given to careful history taking, physical examination, and other less costly procedures that are sufficient to rule out serious disease in the great majority of patients with headache and other neurologic complaints. Use of the CT scanner should be confined to the relatively small proportion of patients in whom there is evidence warranting further diagnostic study. If we fail to exercise this kind of sensible discrimination, we will incur costs far beyond our ability to sustain.

A word should be said about another phenomenon closely related to the technologic imperative: the pressures to increase the supply of physicians. In addition to the belief that more hospitals beds and more technical gadgetry will somehow assure us of being healthier, there is a widely prevalent assumption that the more physicians we have the healthier we will be. On the face of it, this sounds logical; in fact, it is possible to have too many physicians, just as it is possible to have too many CT scanners or too many open-heart surgery units. An excess of physicians tends to cause unnecessary hospitalization and unnecessary surgery. Fuchs and Kramer note that "supply factors (technology and number of physicians) appear to be of decisive importance in determining the utilization of and expenditures for physicians' services."[10] Despite continued demands by some for the creation of new medical schools, I believe that increasing the supply of physicians will have a direct (and unfavorable) impact upon total expenditures for health care, but relatively little, if any, demonstrable impact upon health status.

Depersonalization of Medical Care

Perhaps the most widely discussed and universally deplored characteristic of medical care today is its depersonalization. This is usually contrasted very unfavorably with the "one-to-one" relationship between patient and family physician that characterized a good deal of medical practice before World War II. That such depersonalization exists and that it is unfortunate are widely shared conclusions. Its causes are not simply the fault of "modern technology" but rather a complex set of interrelated factors. Most of these factors made their appearance in a significant way in the early 1940s and gained rapid momentum in the post-World War II era.

Specialization is a major element in this picture. It has become increasingly unlikely that any single practitioner will care for all the needs of any one patient. Furthermore, it is unlikely that any practitioner will have the competence to understand fully what is being done for that patient by the variety of specialists who participate in his or her care. Moreover, each specialist tends to be preoccupied with the increasingly complex technology within his or her own area of practice. Specialists are correspondingly less willing (or able) to attend to the needs of the "whole patient."

Another element is the increasing dependence upon technology in communication between patient and physician. Telephone contact, including telephone diagnosis and treatment, has become more and more accepted as a part of the medical care process. In addition, many physicians now utilize printed history forms, to be self-administered by their patients, as a supplement to the direct exchange of information between patient and physician. (It does not take much imagination to visualize, in the brave new world of tomorrow, that the printed, self-administered history form will give way to a cathode ray tube display as an interface between patient and computer.)

Physicians are increasingly dependent upon technology for the making of diagnoses (laboratory, x-ray, CT scanning, and so on), and are relying less and less upon the careful taking of history and the skillful performance of physical diagnosis. There is less conversation between patient and physician, and less physical contact. As such skills are used less frequently, they are taught less intensively; fewer medical students are interested in learning these skills, and, indeed, fewer physicians are able to teach them.

In turn, these various trends accelerated the one overall trend that perhaps best epitomizes the technologic wave that has swept American medicine in the second half of the 20th century: the increasing dominance of the hospital as the locus of medical care. Partly because of its size, partly because of its ability to attract philanthropic gifts and, most importantly, because of the impact of third-party reimbursement, the hospital has been the one agent most able to mobilize the capital resources necessary to acquire the incredibly expensive technologic gadgetry that accompanied the scientific explosion in medicine. In the modern hospital environment, the patient feels most acutely the impersonal quality of machine-mediated care.

Diseases and Disorders Resulting from the Use of Technology

A significant and disturbing consequence of modern technology has been the occurrence of diseases or abnormal conditions whose cause can be traced to the technology itself. Occurrence of diseases caused by physicians has long been recognized with such disorders being characterized as iatrogenic (doctor-generated). A classic example is the patient who constantly seeks to protect himself against cardiac strain because of an excessive fear of damaging his heart, resulting from overzealous warnings by his physician. This patient may stop exercising, playing games or engaging in any activity requiring a little exertion.

At almost every stage of the medical care process, a growing role is played by machines. An increasing variety of illnesses and disorders can be traced in whole or in part to the use of the machine themselves, a panoply of "technogenic" diseases. Transfusion reactions can be caused by the administration of blood that has been improperly matched. In a literal sense, such episodes are the result of human error. But, they never could have occurred in the absence of the technologic developments that made it possible (and necessary) to administer blood transfusions so commonly.

Potential deleterious effects from the use of mammography in screening for breast cancer are the subject of major controversy. Any x-ray exposure produces some risk of causing cancer. Exposure in mammography is very small, and new techniques offer the promise of even further reduction in exposure. But some experts believe that the number of breast cancer cases that may be *produced* among women screened by mammography techniques will be greater than the number of cases of cancer *detected* through the screening process.

Use of recently developed techniques for fetal monitoring in utero has enabled obstetricians to identify the occurrence of fetal distress at an earlier stage than would otherwise be possible. This permits the obstetrician to intervene in the course of labor and save the life of the baby. Although originally perceived as having major value in high-risk births, fetal monitoring has been used increasingly on a routine basis during the past decade. During the same period of time the rate of caesarean section has more than doubled, bringing with it potential hazards for the mother, as well as substantial cost increases. There is a serious difference of opinion among obstetricians as to whether this increased rate is justifiable, or whether it is due, at least in part, to overenthusiastic application of fetal monitoring with some undesirable consequences. The majority viewpoint apparently endorses the widespread use of monitoring and the associated increase in caesarean sections.[11] Some authorities, however, have raised important questions about the true impact of the new technology.[12] Despite a marked increase in the caesarean section rate among electronically monitored patients, they concluded that there is not a demonstrable improvement in perinatal outcome.[13]

Merely being admitted to a hospital exposes one to the risk of acquiring an infection from the hospital environment. It has been estimated that 5 percent all hospital admissions in this country will be complicated by such infections, and that 15,000 patients die annually as a result.[14]

Laboratory errors may result in unnecessary or even harmful therapeutic actions. More often than not, incorrect laboratory results are caused by human error rather than "technologic error." Yet, it is the growth of laboratory technology as a whole that has resulted in an overwhelming increase in the number of laboratory procedures and unprecedented dependence upon laboratory findings to establish diagnoses. This, in turn, has created the conditions under which increased numbers of errors inevitably will occur.

Clearly, technologic progress is a mixed blessing. Every technologic advance and every increase in the extent to which technology is applied in the medical care process has brought with it significant hazards which work to the detriment of patients.

Some Special Dilemmas

Some of the advantages and disadvantages associated with the growing application of technology to medical care have been identified. Many of these are important and have very substantial impact, for better or worse. Some of the most difficult issues raised by the application of technology to medicine, however, do not lend themselves readily to classification as "desirable" or "undesirable" results. Complex social, legal, economic, ethical, and philosophic values are involved.

In many instances the dilemmas themselves are quite evident although the solutions are not. Views as to the appropriate solutions vary widely. It is not my purpose to express a personal judgment about these various matters, nor even to discuss them in detail, but merely to identify a few salient issues.

For many years, the ability to terminate pregnancy with virtually negligible hazard to the life or physical health of a pregnant woman has provoked heated controversy. At issue is not only the biologic question of when life begins, but also complex legal questions and exquisitely sensitive religious and moral ones.

At the opposite end of the life scale, technology has confronted us with questions regarding the prolongation of life beyond the point when an individual (and his or her family) may wish it to be prolonged. Indeed, life-sustaining technology has enabled us to maintain some vital functions after other functions apparently have disappeared. Technology has brought us to the point where we cannot always determine whether an individual whose cardiac, respiratory, and kidney functions we are maintaining can actually be said with certainty to be alive.

In between these extremes, we have the technical capability to provide artificial kidney functioning for an individual who would otherwise die. With such assistance, this individual can maintain a very significant degree of effective biologic and social functioning. Some patients find the techniques of kidney dialysis and the life style it imposes to be so distasteful that they expressed a preference for dying. Under such conditions, should the patient be permitted to order the discontinuance of kidney dialysis and to die? Different questions arise with reference to the great majority of patients on kidney dialysis who wish to continue with the procedure: How much can our society afford in order to keep one patient alive? Is $25,000 a year a reasonable expenditure for such a purpose? In the United States today we are spending approximately $1 billion to maintain approximately 40,000 patients on kidney dialysis. If we deem this expenditure to be appropriate, are we willing to spend $2 billion annually to provide such care for 80,000 patients (the number currently estimated as the maximum for whom kidney dialysis might be required at current population levels)? What judgment would be made if some new technology were developed which, at a cost of $24,000 per patient per annum, would extend the lives of 600,000 patients who die annually of heart disease? Would we foot the bill for an additional $15 billion annually? Should we limit such technology only to patients whose lives probably would be extended by at least two years? Or one year? Or should the technology be applied, at the same $25,000 price tag, even to a patient whose life would be extended by only a few months? What other goods or services would we be willing to forego in order to be able to commit $15 billion dollars for this purpose?

Does genetic research, that is, recombinant DNA technology, involve the possibility of creating new forms of life that would pose significant hazards for human beings? How great is that risk? Experts disagree. How are we to know whom to believe?

If we soon are to develop the ability to clone human life, that is, to produce perfect replicas of existing individuals, should we proceed to do so? Should everyone be entitled to avail himself or herself of such incredible technology? How should the rules be set, and by whom?

Concluding Thoughts

Technology clearly is a mixed blessing for human beings in medicine as in so many other fields. In cases where we have attained fundamental understanding of disease processes, we have been able to develop preventive and curative measures that have greatly decreased the burden of diseases upon the human race, often at relatively low cost and with a few or no deleterious effects. Limited knowledge, on the other hand, has produced extraordinarily costly solutions that are temporary in nature, accompanied by unexpected and unwanted side effects which are unpleasant, frequently harmful, occasionally fatal.

Rapid growth of technology has been associated with an increasing dependence upon machines and an increasing depersonalization of the medical transactions between patient and physician. Individuals and families can do much more to enhance and maintain their own health than most of us seem willing to do. Many of us are the victims of "overdoctoring": overdiagnosis, overtreatment, and overhospitalization. Our tendency is to abuse our health and then turn to physicians to "bail us out." Physicians tend to apply the full array of diagnostic and therapeutic tools in every instance and this simply does not make sense.

As the complexity of our technology has grown, its costs have grown. We now find that the burden of delivering medical care has reached the point where our national economy is under serious pressure. Stated succinctly, we know how to do more things than we can afford. We even know how to do more things than some of us want to do, or want to have done to us.

Advances of technology have raised problems of the most extraordinary complexity for all of us in medical care as in other aspects of society. Does the unlimited application of medical technology offer significant social and human benefits? Will our most important social and human values be better served by placing limits on the resources we commit to medical care and by deploying some of our resources elsewhere?

Many people have indicated their concern with these complex problems. It is vital that the solutions not be left to the professionals alone. Dr. Edmund Pellegrino[15] has stated the issue eloquently:

> Crucial to any genuine conception of a democratic society is the guarantee that its members ultimately shall decide what is good

> for the whole. Anything less, no matter how benignly intended, is paternalism at best and tyranny at worst. In a technological society, the potential for tyranny lies as much in the power of expert knowledge as in politics or police force.

Hopefully, people will be stimulated to consider their own viewpoints on how technology affects fundamental issues of sickness and health. Thought should be given to the objectives of medical care, the organization of the health care industry, the functions of the various health professionals, and the nature of the interactions between members of those professions and the people whom they serve.

References

1. Faxon, N. W. A history of hospitals. In E. D. Bachmeyer & G. Hartment (Eds.), *The hospital in modern society.* New York: The Commonwealth Fund, 1943.
2. Haagensen, C. D., & Lloyd, W. E. D. *A hundred years of medicine.* New York: Sheridan House, 1943.
3. McKeown, T. Determinants of health. *Human Nature,* 1978 *1* (4), 60–67.
4. Banta, H. D., & Sanes, J. R. Assessing the social impacts of medical technologies. *Journal of Community Health,* 1978, *3,* 245–258.
5. Thomas, L. Commentary: The future impact of science and technology on medicine. *BioScience,* 1974, *24,* 99–105.
6. Altman, L. K., Study backs only seven days in hospital for some heart attack victims. *The New York Times,* February 3, 1978.
7. McNerney, W. *The role of technology in the development of health institution goals and programs.* Paper presented to HEW Conference on Technology and Health Care Systems. San Francisco, January 20, 1972.
8. Shabecoff, P. Soaring price of medical care puts a serious strain on economy. *The New York Times,* May 7, 1978.
9. White, K. L. Health problems and priorities and the health professions (Editorial). *Preventive Medicine,* 1977, *6,* 560–566.
10. Fuchs, V. R., & Kramer, M. J. *Determinants of expenditures for physicians' services in the U.S., 1948–68.* DHEW Publication No. (HSM) 73–3013, December 1972.

11. Shenker, L., Post, R. C. & Seiler, J. S. Routine electronic monitoring of fetal heart rate and uterine activity during labor. *Obstetrics and Gynecology.* 1975, *46,* 185–189.
12. Miller, C. A. *The unexplained increase in caesarean section rates.* Unpublished, 1977.
13. Haverkamp, A. D., et al. The evaluation of continuous fetal heart rate monitoring in high-risk pregnancy. *American Journal of Obstetrics and Gynecology,* 1976, *125,* 310.
14. Health professionals seek to avert risk of hospital-related infections. *The New York Times,* June 5, 1978.
15. Pellegrino, E. D., Decision-making in a technologic society (Editorial). *The Pharos,* 1978, *41* (1), 33.

Chapter 3

A BETTER LIFE THROUGH MEDICAL TECHNOLOGY

Con: Identifying the Issues for Debate

Michael M. Stewart

Conceptual Analysis

In this discussion, I have been asked to defend the following proposition:

> Medical technology has done little to improve health, life expectancy, and the quality of life. Social and economic advances have made more of an impact and will continue to do so in the future.

This task is difficult for several reasons. Many points have been already covered by others in lucid and thorough presentations. Second, I am not a radical disbeliever in medical technology. Indeed, it would be difficult to be a physician actively involved in direct patient care if I truly believe that medical technology had little or no use. My chief difficulty, however, is that the thesis which I am asked to defend is unclear and requires some conceptual analysis before we can proceed with any useful discussion.

It is interesting and symbolic that a general internist with a special interest in primary care and community medicine has been asked to take the antitechnology line, while a surgeon involved with critical care is defending the opposite viewpoint. A debate is thus seemingly posed between a proponent of technology-intensive, dramatic one-on-one life-saving techniques for patient rescue and a socially-conscious primary care clinician who deals with everyday medical problems and their relations to cultural, behavioral, and economic factors. I prefer, however, to view this debate as a process of exploration. Both sides of the argument must be developed in more carefully refined terms so that areas of agreement and areas of controversy can be mapped out carefully.

A most critical issue in this debate is to separate areas of disagreement about *facts* from areas of disagreement about *values.* A second important issue is to separate disagreements about proven facts from disagreements about *expectations, predictions,* and *hypotheses.* In short, we really cannot, and should not, engage in a serious debate until we have reached a general level of agreement about the range and types of positive impacts that medical technology has had and can have on health status, what types of decisions we are likely to face regarding further development and deployment of medical technology in the future, and what are the expected costs, benefits and trade-offs that will have to be considered in such decisions.

A major decision in which the active consumer is likely to participate is regarding the allocation of scarce health care resources for expensive diagnostic and/or therapeutic medical equipment. While the technical details of medical tools and procedures are certainly complex, the diligent consumer should at least be able to determine the general purposes, major applications, and likely risks of a new medical technology to a sufficient degree to participate in the decision-making process. Perhaps the most important thing for the participating consumer to understand is the decision-making process itself. There is no better way to appreciate this process than to experience it first-hand, but it can be usefully sketched out.

In order to make a decision, there must be at least two alternatives to choose from. Each alternative has two major components, the expected outcome of the decision and the value attached to that outcome. There is almost always a substantial degree of uncertainty about the likelihood of any specific outcome actually taking place. Thus, the outcomes of possible decisions are commonly stated in terms of probabilities: for example, if we decide to do *X*, there is a 50 percent probability that *Y* will happen, whereas if we decide to do *P*, there is only a 25 percent probability that *Q* will happen. Action *X* may cost $1000 and action *P* $750; then there must be careful consideration of which result, *Y* or *Q*, is more highly valued. Here is where the decision-making process often becomes most complex and controversial. There may not be agreement or consensus on the relative values assigned to these two expected outcomes. Even more important, it may not be at all clear just how a group of decision makers should reach such an agreement or consensus when value differences occur. Some people would say that this is where the health planning process becomes frankly political. That is certainly true enough if what we mean is a participatory process where there is a commitment to working out disagreements in order to arrive at an acceptable course of action. However, it is critically important that consumers participating in decisions on health care continually try to make distinctions. Disagreements may occur over the expected probability that certain outcomes will follow from certain decisions. In comparison, disagreements may also occur over the value or benefit that is assigned to these expected outcomes, if they do indeed occur.

What Are the Basic Issues of the Debate?

When I said that the basic proposition which I am asked to defend is an unclear one, it was for two reasons. First, the proposition includes two statements: that medical technology is relatively ineffective and that socioeconomic advances have had a greater health impact. These statements are not logically connected and really deserve to be examined separately. Second, both statements should be analyzed in terms of both facts and values.

An ever growing body of evidence could be mustered to defend or refute either of these two assertions. One way to approach the subject would be to argue that advances in medical technology usually go hand in hand with general socioeconomic advances. Societies usually do not experience one type of advance without the other, thus the entire discussion is spurious. In addition to being cynical, this approach is manifestly not true with regard to many communities in the United States, particularly in the inner city. There are well-documented examples of advanced medical technology being introduced into communities which are not yet receiving minimally adequate levels of basic medical care and other social services. There are also an increasing number of situations, particularly in Europe, where general socioeconomic advances—in education, housing, unemployment policy, and pension arrangements, for example—are quite widespread, but where additional investment in expensive medical technology is consciously being rationed in the public sector. What emerges is a fundamental social question: To what degree whould further societal investment in costly medical technology be given explicit preference over investment in other areas of social welfare? There are many practical decisions as well as policy issues to be resolved concerning this question.

Another approach would be to construct an antitechnology ideology in order to argue that medical technology does not exert an effective influence on health status. Medical specialists, taken in the aggregate, are part of the technocratic establishment, motivated primarily by economic motives and likely to induce medical problems as quickly as they ameliorate them. In this line of thinking, surgery is practiced to excess, leading to unnecessary complications, more drugs, more surgery, and of course greater costs. Use of new and ever more powerful drugs causes adverse reactions, more visits to doctors, and sometimes more hospital admissions and even more patient deaths. There can be no doubt that all therapeutic interventions entail measurable degrees of risk for patients. The phenomenon of iatrogenesis (physician-induced illness) is a problem of increasing concern. Yet, the risks and hazards of modern medical interventions will best be dealt with not by blanket condemnation, but rather by careful quantitative analysis of the effectiveness of each specific type of medical intervention. An important example of this analytic approach is the recent book by Bunker and his colleagues[1] on the costs, risks, and benefits of surgery. While the technical details of this book make parts of it difficult reading for the consumer, it illustrates an important approach based on a search for the appropriate facts, rather than relying on ideology, intuition, or preconception. It also gives an excellent presentation of the complex process of medical decision making in the application of sophisticated technology.

To get at the basic issues underlying the proposition which I have been asked to defend, however, the most reasonable approach is to ask whether we have all agreed on what we mean by medical technology, whether we have sound evidence of the actual impact of any specific new technology on health status, and whether there is good evidence of nontechnologic impact on health status during the same time period. There is a rapidly growing literature on specific medical technologies. Informed health consumers should not only be aware of major publications in this field, but indeed should find a way to be carefully advised about what to read in order to continue to be well-informed.[2-4]

I want to be quite clear that I am not opposed in principle nor on ideologic grounds to the proper application of the most sophisticated technology available. I recently followed a patient whose brain tumor was diagnosed and successfully treated only after an extraordinarily thorough evaluation including brain scans, CAT scans, multiple biopsies, and extirpative neurosurgery. I am impressed with the neurosurgical armamentarium. I do have, however, some serious reservations as to whether enthusiastic proponents of expensive, equipment-intensive modern medical technology have adequately weighed the relative costs and expected benefits (financial and other) of all the available options. Indeed, were the proponents really in a position to do so? Understandably, the radiologist or surgeon with a new technique wants to apply it if it is thought to be effective. If the technology is both self-amortized and reimbursed by major third-party payers, why not? One answer is that every new technology that is woven onto our "routine" health care system ends up costing all of us a considerable amount. So-called advances in health and medical care delivery should not be slipped into place without a fair public hearing as to the anticipated costs, expected benefits, the degree of possible risk to patients, and the criteria by which effectiveness and impact are to be evaluated.

Why not say the protechnologists? Why should cost be a limiting factor? Isn't health too important an issue to turn over to cost accountants? When I encounter this argument, I usually feel compelled to point out that the most expensive medical technology is not preventive, and often not even curative; that it is readily available to only a limited number of persons; and that the health budget may grow a bit more, but it will always have finite limits. Resources will always be less than optimal. We will always have to make choices.

What Are the Objectives of Health Care?

Health care systems are increasingly difficult to separate from other spheres of society. Victor Fuchs[5] noted three basic points of view in what he called the economist's view of the world: resources are scarce, resources have alternative uses, and that different persons have different wants and preferences. Obviously, it is incumbent on the proponents of wider use of sophisticated medical technology to be familiar with the extent of available resources in the health care sector, with their feasible alternative uses, and perhaps most importantly, with the relative preferences or values of those for whom these increasingly scarce resources are purportedly being expended. For example, suppose that in a given health care setting, there is a finite and fixed amount of money in the budget to initiate new programs. Two feasible alternatives are to improve maternal care services by identifying high risk mothers early in pregnancy and provide necessary consultations; and expand neonatal services for low birthweight infants, including aggressive nutritional supplementation efforts.

Admittedly, both maternal and neonatal services should be improved if resources permitted. However, if a choice had to be made between these two different types of activities as relative priorities, which one should receive a higher priority? What is more "important," reduction of the maternal mortality rate, or reduction of the neonatal and infant mortality rate? Can reduction of these two rates be measured on the same scale? Is there any reasonable way to make such a choice? Is it, in fact, necessary to make such a choice?

These questions are not idle ones; such decisions are being made daily. It is clear that the issues of values and facts, of expected outcomes and the importance attached to these expected outcomes, are central in the decision-making process.

How Should Medical Technology Be Assessed?

Broadly defined, medical technology includes a wide array of techniques, drugs, equipment, and procedures that are used by health professionals for a variety of purposes, including diagnosis, therapy, rehabilitation, and prevention, as well as for the administration and management of health and medical care resources and services. In this broad sense, "medical technology" is virtually equivalent to "the health and medical care system." Therefore, to question the effectiveness of medical technology is the same as asking whether the existing health care system "works." Important questions to be asked are: How good is the evidence that medical technology is actually responsible for reducing morbidity and mortality? Are the results worth the costs? Discussion of these basic questions must be presented in terms of medical technology's "efficacy" (or "effectiveness") on the one hand, versus its "cost-effectiveness" on the other hand.

The record of the past 100 years suggests that a distinction is warranted among the following types of technologies: public health, simple medical care, complex medical care, and nonmedical technologies. An example of a public health technology would be the introduction of clean water in the late 19th century, and more recently, fluoridation of public water sources. A simple medical technology would be tetanus immunization, or the treatment of strep throat with penicillin. A complex medical technology would be open-heart surgery or coronary bypass. A nonmedical technology reflecting socioeconomic factors would be public television's impact on the nation's children in terms of its effect on health beliefs and health care utilization.

There is considerable evidence to suggest that simpler medical technologies are more effective than complex technolgies, when measured in overall social terms. On the other hand, complex technologies tend to be applied narrowly to selected patient groups. Moreover, complex medical technologies tend to become self-perpetuating. It is important to distinguish between the sometimes competing goals of refining technology with the notion of generalizing its application, and refining technology for the purpose of better serving the limited patient group for whom the application of a specific technology was originally intended or for whom it is most obviously beneficial.

SUMMARY

Pro- and antitechnology arguments notwithstanding, the health care consumer who wishes to play an active and constructively critical role in decision making in the health care field has a responsibility to be well-informed regarding the facts of new medical technologies. Even more important is the consumer's obligation to understand the decision-making process regarding the allocation of scarce societal resources for a finite set of social objectives.

References

1. Bunker, J. P., Barnes, B. A., & Mosteller, F., *Costs, risks, and benefits of surgery.* New York: Oxford University Press, 1977.
2. U.S. Congress, Office of Technology Assessment. *Development of medical technology: Opportunities for assessment.* Washington, D.C.: U.S. Government Printing Office, 1976.
3. Institute of Medicine. *A policy statement: Computed tomographic scanning.* Washington, D.C.: National Academy of Sciences, 1977.
4. Egdahl, R. H., & Gertman, P. M. (eds.) *Technology and the quality of health care.* Germantown, Md.: Aspen Systems Corp., 1978.
5. Fuchs, V. R. *Who shall live? Health, economics, and social choice.* New York: Basic Books, 1974.

A BETTER LIFE THROUGH MEDICAL TECHNOLOGY

Pro: The Argument for Medical Technology

Louis R. M. Del Guercio

Resolved: Medical technology has made meaningful contributions to improving health, life expectancy, and the quality of life and will do even better in the future.

Currently, it is popular to denigrate "halfway technology," that apt phrase coined by Lewis Thomas,[1] as one manifestation of a modern life-style that longs for a bucolic simple existence free from the tyranny of the machine. This antitechnology trend has gained remarkable momentum because it seems to offer something for everyone politically. To the liberals, the doctrine implies a central influence over personal behavior to create a better and healthier society free from the costs of devices manufactured by industry and procedures promoted by physicians. To the conservatives, antitechnology means lower taxes and the freedom to purchase whatever life support one can afford.[2] Guilt regarding the critically ill indigent is absolved by the view that the poor bring disease upon themselves by an imprudent life-style. No one has proved that halfway technology can prolong meaningful life anyway.

Thomas' original essay was not a plea to eliminate technical innovation but an argument for fundamental research on the nature of the basic disease process. We still do not know the root cause of heart disease, peptic ulcer, diabetes, kidney disease, and stroke. But with halfway technology alone, the death rates from these problems have been reduced significantly. The National Center for Health Statistics has found a 12 percent drop in death rates for men between the ages of 55 and 64 during the five years ending in 1974. Modern physicians would be paralyzed without access to hemodialysis, pacemakers, respirators, cardiac monitoring, and total parenteral nutrition. More than any other factor, total parenteral nutrition has significantly reduced death rates from severe trauma and burns. Stanley Dudrick[3] of Houston now has a number of patients who survived burns over 90 percent of their body and recovered as a result of his sophisticated nutritional support with maintenance of immune competence and energy reserves. Last year, the *New England Journal of Medicine*[4] ran a lead article describing patient physician "agreements" to abandon therapy in such "hopeless" burn cases. My view is that a society that will spend $25,000 a year maintaining convicted murderers because it will not fully sanction capital punishment will never tolerate euthanasia on so-called hopeless cases. Typical of this attitude is a letter to the editor which appeared in the *New York Times*[5] on May 6, 1978. It was from an accountant who pointed out that the cost to society of his kidney dialysis and two transplants was over $50,000 from age 26, but that his taxes will soon have repaid the cost of keeping him alive. He ended by writing, "I thank God I was born in America."

We cannot afford to coast along on past accomplishments. There already is evidence that this antitechnology trend has cost the United States its lead in research and development. Between 1971 and 1976, patents granted to United States residents declined by 21 percent. Those granted to foreigners grew by 16 percent and became 37 percent of all United States patents granted in 1976. It must be remembered that the CAT scanner, about which there has been so much bureaucratic disagreement, was an American concept but a British development. Artificial hip joints, which have restored over 200,000 patients to painless ambulation, was also a British innovation.

Technology Is Not a Scapegoat

Technology should not be made the scapegoat for the enormous increases in health care costs (110 billion dollars from 1950 to 1976!); 55 percent of the increase was due to inflation and less than 4 percent was attributable to increased technology. Population growth, increased utilization, the malpractice turmoil, and unionization of the health labor force accounted for the rest of the cost explosion. In 1966 the average hospital wage was $4000; in 1976, it was $8650. Hospital malpractice premiums in the millions add from $17 to $25 to the per diem cost of hospitalization. It is estimated by the American Hospital Association that overregulation accounts for 20 percent of hospital costs. In New York State, the average hospital must respond to 164 different agencies; 96 at the state level, 40 at the federal level, and 18 city, country, and voluntary agencies. Costs of this morass of red tape have been documented but *not* the benefits to society.

The only way that society can make advanced medical technology available to all who desire it at a reasonable cost is through the application of cost-lowering technology itself. Feldstein[6] points out that cost-lowering technology is characterized as raising the benefits of inexpensive care proportionately more than the benefits of expensive care. By benefits we mean some combination of increased therapeutic success, reduced diagnostic uncertainty, and increased patient comfort. Examples of cost-lowering technology include ambulatory surgical centers, medical information systems, and effective assessment of preoperative risk.

Medical Information Systems

One of the most promising approaches to cost-lowering technology is the hospital medical information system. A recent report on the cost effectiveness of such a system in use at the El Camino Hospital in Mountainview, California was released by the Battelle Memorial Institute under contract from the National Center for Health Services Research.[7] Developed by the Technicon Corporation, the system is a real time, comprehensive, integrated, medical information network within the hospital which operates from a large-scale computer. It is connected to video and printer terminals located throughout the hospital. Doctors, nurses, and other hospital professional and clerical personnel interact directly with the system through these terminals to enter, retrieve, and print clinical, financial, and administrative information. The system automates a great many of the patient-oriented information processing tasks that are performed thousands of times daily in a hospital. Patient information from the admission through discharge is captured accurately and routed in the most logical and efficient manner. Physicians' medical orders, once entered, are sent to the proper hospital unit for execution and the results verified and recorded. Labor-intensive, cottage industry approaches to hospital practice with their errors and inaccuracies cannot compete with this innovative development. The Battelle report showed that the net cost benefits to El Camino Hospital were $41,000 per month which equalled $4.10 per diem reduction, plus the value of enhanced patient care, reduced hospital stay, and accurate charge capture. I am personally familiar with the Technicon Medical Information System having used it at the Saint Barnabas Medical Center in New Jersey. The increased productivity of the average practitioner caring for patients with such a system is truly remarkable. One wonders why all hospitals are not switching over to this system.

There are two problems with the implementation of similar systems for other hospitals. One, most hospitals have relatively little investment capital and the high start-up and initial costs impose cash-flow problems during the first two or three years that may exceed one million dollars. Second, since savings are passed through to third party reimbursement agencies, there are inadequate financial incentives for hospitals to adopt such systems. Hospitals state that they take the financial risks and get no return on their investment. If the outcome is successful, third-party insurers reap the cost benefits.

Cost-Lowering Technology

There are other examples of the need for cost-lowering technology, one of which involves older people and the determination of surgical risk. By 1985, the over 65 population will have grown by 20 percent. At that time, the elderly will comprise 12 percent of the population. Elderly people use three times more medical care than the national average. They spend $1521 per capita as compared with $550 for the national average. In particular, their surgical mortality rates are much higher than the national average. Recently, the Commission on Professional and Hospital Activities reported on an analysis of some 13 million operations performed during 1974–1975. Overall, the surgical mortality rate for patients over the age of 65 was 4.88 percent. Since the survey included 40 percent of all hospital discharges, extrapolation to the total national level indicates that over 135,000 yearly deaths occur following surgery in the elderly. Aside from the anguish and human misery, the cost of these deaths is enormous, since many patients linger in intensive care units at an average expense of $20,000. Thus, the total national cost of surgical deaths in the elderly is over 2.7 billion dollars. Our work[8] has shown that any operation in an elderly patient carries a high risk and that special methods for the preoperative assessment of the physiologic cardiopulmonary reserve are needed. At present, this approach to the evaluation of risk requires invasive measurements of cardiac function and oxygen uptake in the lung at considerable expense. However, the cost benefits and reduction of mortality are clear. Although physicians and hospital administrators are often criticized for jumping on the bandwagon for every technical innovation, technology transfer in medicine is actually notoriously slow. Our automated physiologic profile for the assessment of operative risk has taken years of sweat to catch on, even in university centers.

Resuscitate Technical Innovation

Rosalyn Yalow,[9] in her 1977 lecture when she received the Nobel Prize in Medicine, supported the view that physicians themselves were the greatest skeptics when it came to new medical technology. Her magnificent technique of radioimmunoassay took 15 years to reach the market place. Now it is used for everything from cancer detection to reducing digitalis toxicity. Another Nobel Laureate, Sir Peter Medawar,[10] deplores this antitechnology trend and calls it medical Luddism after the naive political movement of the early industrial revolution which sought to halt progress by wrecking machines in an attempt to protect hand labor. Sir Peter stated "the fear is rather that mechanized medicine diminishes man by depriving him of the chance of making a dignified (and cheap) exit of the kind that people still alive, believe to be coveted by those on the point of dying."

Medical technical innovation in the United States needs resuscitation. Statements such as the following by Howard Hiatt,[11] Dean of the Harvard School of Public Health have done great harm, "Proof of effectiveness, by itself, cannot justify the spread of costly new technology." Bureaucrats have also imposed stiff and punitive regulations through the Medical Device Amendment of 1976 to the basic Food, Drug and Cosmetic Act. Meeting these regulations will take its heaviest toll on the small manufacturer who in the past has been responsible for such innovations as the artificial kidney, pacemakers, respirators, and most of the other life-saving devices. It used to take 3 years and 3 million dollars to bring a product into the market; overnight, the new regulations have increased this to 5 years and 5 million.

SUMMARY

In summary, medical technology is our only hope for the containment of medical costs and improvement in the quality of care. Technologic entrepreneurs are an endangered species. In the past, these entrepreneurs provided great benefits with very little return on investments in time and effort. The true innovator in the field of medical devices has been overregulated and undersupported. If the technological innovator disappears from the American scene, health care will suffer and we will either do without or import from abroad.

REFERENCES

1. Thomas, L. *The lives of a cell.* New York, The Viking Press, 1974, pp. 31–37.
2. Del Guercio, L. R. M. Oath hasn't been amended, but vigilance is needed. *New York Times* September 2, 1977.
3. Dudrick, S. J. & Long, J. D. Applications and hazards of intravenous hyperalimentation. *Annual Review of Medicine.* 1977, *28:*517–28.
4. Imbus, S. H. & Zawacki, B. E. Autonomy for burned patients when survival is unprecented. *New England Journal of Medicine.* 1977, *297:* 308–311.
5. Raymond, F. J. After the transplant. *New York Times.* May 6, 1978.
6. Feldstein, M. S. *The rising cost of hospital care.* National Center for Health Services Research and Development, Washington, D.C.: Information Resources Press, 1971.

7. Barrett, J. P., Barnum, R. A., Gordon, B. B., & Pesut, R. N. *Evaluation of the implementation of a medical information system in a general community hospital.* Final report, Battelle Columbus Laboratories. Springfield, Va.: NTIS Publication 248340, 1975.
8. Del Guercio, L. R. M. The reduction of surgical mortality. *Cincinnati Journal of Medicine,* 1974, *55,* 145.
9. Yalow, R. S. Radioimmunoassay: A probe for the fine structure of biologic systems. *Science,* 1978, *200,* 1236.
10. Medawar, P. B. Thoughts on progress. *Hospital Practices,* 1976, *11*(10), 107–108.
11. Hiatt, H. H. Too much medical technology? *Wall Street Journal.* June 24, 1976.

Chapter 4

DECISION MAKING: WHO IS THE EXPERT?

Arthur Levin

New Mandates for Consumers

It has only been in the last several years that consumerism has turned its attention to the area of medical care. I assume that part of the reluctance to apply lessons of consumerism learned in other areas resulted from the belief that medical care was "too complex" and "too technical" for consumers to play an important role in shaping policy. That has all changed. Now we have health planning policies that mandate consumer participation in the decision-making process. Indeed, although consumerism may have come late to the medical care field, it is perhaps more firmly required there than elsewhere. Yet, there are still lay people who are reluctant to accept the fact that they can participate with parity in decision making. On the other hand, there are many professionals who believe it unwise and unscientific to allow nonprofessionals to help set policy. This mystique of medicine, science, and technology continues to plague us.

Experts and Consumers

An expert is usually defined as someone having acquired a special skill in or knowledge of a particular subject through professional training *or* practical experience. In recent years, the emphasis has been on professional training as the means through which people become experts and achieve special status. Experts are specialists and authorities. As medicine has become more and more specialized we have, by definition, produced more and more experts; and authorities are persons whose opinions, it is said, *deserve* our acceptance. There is no question that the lay person is confronted by an ever increasing degree of specialization. Often, the consumer may find it convenient to accept the authority and submit willingly to the decisions made by the expert. I am sure, however, that many consumers would be able to testify how dangerous to your health such acceptance of authority can be.

What happened to make consumers take a strong interest in medical care and to insist that participation in decision making and planning be written into law? I believe that when consumers saw the experts differing about increasingly risky and invasive technologies, they decided they had to protect their own health by getting involved. Harsh lessons from birth control pills, DES, thyroid irridation, and mammography screening are clear: consumer beware, and be involved.

When we hear experts disagree so often, how can we be sure we are listening to the "right" expert when a decision has to be made? If they disagree, which experts should set policy and make decisions? Which experts should be ignored? It is crucial for consumers to play a major role in medical care decision making. Consumers can be fairer in listening to all the varying opinions and shaping policy. Vested interests of researchers, hospitals, laboratories, medical equipment manufacturers and suppliers are often in conflict with the vested interest of the consumer, to be healthy at the least possible cost.

Information Monopoly

The medical mystique is breaking down, but not without a battle. These center around the power that experts have over the public by having access to information that the public does not have. Experts can release information in whatever way will best substantiate their position. A monopoly of information crucial to the decision-making process is one way that medical/technological professionals seek to retain power over consumers. George Bernard Shaw[1] said "All professions are conspiracies against the laity." One way to stop the conspiracy, and to shift the locus of power away from the expert and back to the public is to guarantee open access to information that is crucial to the decision-making process. Having information means having the ability to participate with parity in medical care decision-making. Look at the basic encounter in the medical model, the provider–patient encounter. There have been numerous times that a consumer has complained that the doctor did not take the time to explain satisfactorily the diagnosis, the disease, the therapy, the drug, and so on. The professional may have put the question aside by responding that the doctor knows best; or states that its too complex a subject for the patient to be able to understand. Based on this encounter, it is important that consumers demand the right to retain control over the decisions that affect their lives.

Understandable Language Needed

Not only must there be access to information so that consumers can participate in decision making, but information must be made available in a form that will allow a degree of understanding sufficient to the decision-making task at hand. Professionals can monopolize information and gain power by developing jargon which can only be understood by those practicing the same profession. Some experts may claim that these separate languages are scientifically and technically essential. I believe that their major importance is in helping professionals maintain their dominance over lay people.

Critical Attitude Needed

Development of a questioning and critical attitude is another way in which consumers can protect themselves from the potential dominance of medical experts. Consumers must understand that one expert's opinion can be the opposite of another, equally well trained and credentialled expert. Therefore, a critical and questioning consumer is an important protection from harm. More important than government regulation and peer review in improving the quality of medical care is a consumer that asks questions and assumes that what the expert is saying is not true until proven true. It is here that the mystique of expert authority rears its head again. Many lay people find it difficult to believe that they have the ability to understand a complex problem and to question the professional. It is important for consumers to overcome this timidity and to begin to believe in themselves.

Advisor Role for Professionals

Properly, the role of the specialist is that of advisor to the consumer. Physicians, for example, should be medical advisors to the lay people who would use that information as but one part of the decision-making process about health issues. At present, most professional–lay encounters result in the dominance of the professional. One of the most important changes that can come about in health care is for consumers and professionals to assume new roles; the locus of power should be with the consumer and not with the professional. Experts can also serve as translators for the consumer, that is, taking technical details and rendering them understandable to the nontechnically trained. As mentioned, professionals are reluctant to perform this task. But if medical care providers want to reverse what I see as a steadily worsening relationship with their clients, acceptance of the role of technical advisor might restore these relationships to good health.

Very specialized, highly technical information will always be presented by professionals in the decision-making process. Consumers must be sure to understand the particular bias that each professional has; that is, the consumer must always ask what is the self-interest of the expert. Surgeons recommend surgery, other specialists prefer medical solutions. Consumers must make every effort to seek out different expert opinions to try to confirm or refute the conclusions presented. Even more important is the need for the consumer to follow up on any hint of expert disagreement, particularly on viewpoints which appear to be presented as beyond question.

Government's Role

If the proper role of the professional is that of technical advisor to the consumer, what should be the role of government? As I have already suggested, one role of government should be guaranteeing that the public have open, complete access to the technological information that may affect their well-being through the decision-making process. Government should also insure that such information is presented in a form which is understandable to lay people. Government can also try to make sure that all shades of expert opinion are available in public decision-making. Areas of controversy should be held up for public scrutiny and not hidden from view.

Consumers' Role

A consumer's role in decision making is that of "expert" generalist. On an individual basis this means that consumers must educate themselves about those medical/health issues that concern them. Learning basic facts, asking critically relevant questions, assuming leadership in the decision-making process are all ways to help redefine the relationship of expert and consumer. For those consumers that participate in health planning and health policy decision making, the process is the same, but there is more homework to be done.

Therefore, to answer the question, "Decision making, who is the expert?" I would answer that the expert is the consumer-generalist in whom ultimate power should be vested. The professional-specialist's proper role should be that of advisor and translator. Government should insure that both can perform their respective tasks adequately.

Opportunities exist for consumers to learn how to exercise the new "expert" role most intelligently. Consumers can be taught how to obtain information and to know what is required when deliberating on a specific medical technology issue. Questions can be examined that need to be asked of and answered by expert specialists in their advisory capacity. Consumers can learn how to evaluate the responses. Various consumer-oriented groups offer training and hands-on activities where lay people can acquire practical experience and the stimulation to continue to learn special skills or knowledge in a particular area. Consumers who combine these lessons with good common sense should all be able to become experts.

Reference

1. Shaw, G. B. *The Doctor's Dilemma.* New York: Penguin Books, 1975.

DECISION MAKING: WHO IS THE EXPERT?

Harold L. Light

One of my difficulties stemmed from the fact that the title "Decision Making: Who is The Expert?" suggests that there is an inherent adversary relationship between the health-care provider and the health-care consumer as it relates to the use of medical technology. I do not believe that such a conflict exists. I do believe that the decision-making responsibility about the use of such technology—except in the case of life and death emergencies—does rest, and has always rested with the consumer or his surrogate. In the future, the consumer will be even more assertively involved in the decision-making process about his own health care. Factually, consumers may have abrogated this responsibility in the past. However, that is no reason to suggest that the professional ursurped responsibilities he had no right to assume in the first place or that he usurped the prerogative of the patient in making decisions relating to his own life.

I do not know if my feelings on this subject parallel those of other providers or professionals. It may well be that the basic reason for my feeling as I do on this subject stems from the fact that I am, by training, a social worker and not a hospital administrator. One of the basic principles of social work education is that individuals, in our form of democratic society, have the absolute right of self-determination. This is a principle in which I firmly believe. This basic right pertains in all areas of the individual's functioning and clearly applies in the area of health care. Some of the basic decisions individuals have to make about themselves can, and very often are, essential to their continued health and well being.

Physician Mystique Influences Decisions

Why then should such a discussion take place today? Why would it be assumed that a hospital administrator would necessarily take the position that the health care provider is the expert who should be making the decisions about the use of medical technology? I can only assume that this attitude stems from prior history and a previously existing climate. Health care professionals use the mystique that for years surrounded their role and function. In addition to the mystique, professionals use the authority vested in them by government and by other members of the staff at the hospital at which they happen to be practicing. Very often, this resulted in professionals acting as the omniscient, omnipotent God-like figures some of us came to know in our earlier years.

In the past, higher education was not nearly so universal a phenomenon as it is today. Physicians were seen not only as healers and relievers of pain, but as cultured and learned men. Their knowledge of many things entitled them to make suggestions which, rightly or wrongly, were often accepted by the patient or his family as decisions made for them. Transferential elements in the doctor–patient relationship, plus the factors cited previously, combined with a generally prevailing societal respect for authority. Often, this combination resulted in situations where it appeared as if the patient was not a participant in the decision-making process. I suppose that in many instances, particularly as this relates to the indigent population, decisions were made for the patient without his or her active participation in the process.

Today, we are clearly living in a different era. Authority is a much more elusive element and is as often challenged as accepted. Civil liberties of individuals are much more respected and protected than they were previously. Medicolegal complications have created problems for the modern-day practice of medicine. All these factors serve to ensure that the patient is a much more active participant in the decision-making process relative to his own care.

Surgical Decisions

Several cases, which have received wide publicity in the media in the recent past, characterize the manner in which society, as a whole, and health care institutions, in particular, are now dealing with the question of the impact of medical technology. One such recent well-publicized case in New York City involved a down-and-out Bowery alcoholic who refused to have his gangrenous leg amputated in the face of such a recommendation by the physicians taking care of him. It is not inconceivable that 20 or 30 years ago such an individual would have had his leg amputated, possibly even against his will. This could have taken place because the doctor felt that this was the only way to stop the spread of gangrene and the only way to ultimately preserve the man's life. In today's climate, there is no question in anyone's mind that the physicians who wanted to perform such an amputation would not do so, or even consider the prospects of doing so, against the man's will. Physicians would seek a court order adjudicating the man's incompetence to render a decision in his own behalf. Since such a court order was not forthcoming, the man was allowed to remain in the hospital without having to submit to the surgery in question.

JEHOVAH'S WITNESSES DECISIONS

A somewhat less dramatic and by now less controversial and more frequently occurring situation involves the treatment of Jehovah's Witnesses in hospitals. Courts have always upheld the hospital's responsibility to administer blood or blood derivatives if these prove to be necessary during the course of an infant's hospital stay. Despite this fact, this is never done as a routine, pro forma activity in situations involving the children of Jehovah's Witnesses. In every instance that I know of, the hospitals are required to petition the courts and to get the court's approval to proceed. This procedure is followed regardless of the fact that there is already ample precedent and weight of evidence as to the way parents will respond when the courts order the hospitals to administer such blood products. On the other hand, adults who are Jehovah's Witnesses have increasingly been given the right to make determinations for themselves as to whether they will or will not be provided with blood if that proves to be necessary during the course of a hospital procedure. Of course, no one can say for certain how the courts would react if a physician, acting in good faith and following the precepts of the ethics of this profession, administered blood to a Jehovah's Witness against a previously stated request. Frankly I would find it hard to believe that heavy damages could be inflicted against such a physician. To the best of my knowledge, the situation has never arisen and, considering the trend we are seeing in the health care field in the recent past, it is unlikely to happen.

HEROIC MEASURES DECISIONS

In countless cases, the courts have also held for the patient's right to insist that no "heroic measures" be taken in his behalf for the sake of preserving life beyond the point when life would otherwise cease to exist by most laymen's standards.

Thus, a patient riddled with cancer may chose to advise his physician that he wants no heroic measure taken in the event that he suffers a cardiac arrest. Yet, medical technology, in the forms of defibrillation, may exist to resuscitate such an individual. Similarly, the courts have determined that a terminal cancer patient has the absolute right to refuse treatment for the disease itself. Instead, the patient may choose to be administered to only for the sake of being relieved of the pain attendant to such a terminal condition.

Comatose Patients

Perhaps the most notorious case known to us in recent years and which is, to this very day, with us, is the Karen Quinlan case. This is not the first such case in medical history, nor is it likely to be the last while society debates the moral and ethical issues surrounding the maintenance of life. Through the use of mechanical apparatus, the patient is kept alive while electroencephalograms reveal a flat reading or what has come to be called "brain death." There is no doubt in my mind that a number of people are of the opinion that someone should have "pulled the plug" on Karen Quinlan, as harsh and cruel as that may sound. There is also no doubt in my mind that the plug has been pulled on a number of other patients in similar circumstances. In all likelihood there was an agreement between the patient's family and the professionals responsible for that patient's care. It is surely not for me to pass judgment upon the correctness or incorrectness of such actions. I cite those instances merely to suggest that I know of no circumstances where the professional made that decision by himself. Professionals do not play God in the face of even the remotest suggestion that the patient or his family would have been displeased by such an action.

PHYSICIANS UNFAIRLY MALIGNED

Medical professionals are far from perfect in many respects and may even deserve some of the negative press to which they are now being subjected. My own sense, however, is clearly that the medical profession has been unfairly maligned in the area of patient's rights and in their respect for those rights. If the profession is guilty of anything in this regard, it is probably in not adequately recognizing the degree to which even the strongest individual is thrust into a dependent state by virtue of his need for hospitalization and his need for the resources provided by a hospital and its professionals. Greater sensitivity to the patient's readiness to abrogate his own decision-making responsibility in such a climate would do much to ensure informed consent when such consent is indicated and refusal for treatment when the individual is aware of the potential consequences of such refusal. When most health care providers are so sensitized to their patient's needs and rights, they will find their own work and decision-making process to be less burdensome, their medicolegal exposure to be diminished significantly and their status in the community enhanced. Perhaps even to a level previously held by health care providers in the "good old days."

Chapter 5

WORKSHOP SUMMARIES

Workshop 1: What Consumers Should Know About Evaluating Medical Technology

Moderator: Marcia Pinkett-Heller, M.P.H.
Director, Consumer Education Program
Columbia University School of Public Health
New York, N.Y.

Panelists: Zita Fearon
Chairperson, Consumer Council to the New York City Health Department

Lloyd Novick, M.D.
Deputy Commissioner of Health
New York, N.Y.

Panelists and the moderator raised general social, medical, and economic issues associated with the increasing technology in health care. In addition, they outlined the specific methodologies most commonly used in judging the quality and efficacy of individual practitioners and health facilities.

One of the unforeseen but most interesting issues raised was the question of just what was meant by a "consumer" evaluation. Dr. Novick made a distinction between the concerns of consumers and providers as evaluators. Consumers' concerns were portrayed as primarily subjective (having to do with the "amenities" of care) or involved with those issues pertinent to choosing physicians and facilities with good reputations. He described providers as the objective assessors of health care, via outcome analyses, process reviews, and the application of structural criteria. These procedures were outlined in detail.

Consumer participants, along with panelist Fearon, joined the issue by pointing to the difference between consumers as patients and as board members and planners. Clearly, the workshop participants were there in their role as board members and planners. They wished to familiarize themselves with the standards used by providers in evaluating technology (and all aspects of the system). In addition, the consumers wanted to develop their own criteria of assessing the merits and necessity for specific technologies. Ms. Fearon saw consumers as having to "evaluate the evaluators." Consumers do this by familarizing themselves with those questions which must be asked to determine the quality and efficacy of health services, technologic and otherwise. Furthermore, consumers evaluate evaluators by acting in their official capacities to ensure that all necessary evaluations are performed thoroughly and responsibly.

WORKSHOP 2: PATIENTS' RIGHTS AND INFORMED CONSENT IN A TECHNOLOGIC ERA

Moderator: Mary Robinson
Bronx Borough Coordinator
Health Systems Agency of New York City

Panelists: Sylvia Law, J.D.
Associate Professor
New York University Law School
New York, N.Y.

Enoch Gordis, M.D.
Associate Professor of Medicine
Mt. Sinai School of Medicine
New York, N.Y.

This workshop opened with presentations by the panelists on the subject of informed consent. Professor Law gave a brief history of the doctor's legal obligation to inform patients of the potential risks of medical procedures. She noted a recent shift toward general community standards and away from a strictly professional standard in determining whether a patient has been reasonably informed. Dr. Gordis spoke to the same issues, giving examples from his own practice illustrating a physician's point of view on the complexities of the question of when and how much to inform patients.

A question-and-answer session between the audience and panel members brought up a number of specific problems on this topic. One of the topics concerned the rights of the patient in cases of "ghost surgery," that is, when surgical residents, unbeknownst to the patient, perform operations in place of the "official" surgeon of record. A discussion ensued on the conflict between the rights of individual patients and the need of a teaching institution to train future surgeons. The related question of whether the less affluent or minorities were more likely to become "training subjects" was also raised in this context.

A heated discussion ensued over how thoroughly physicians were obliged to inform their patients of the purposes and risks of medical procedures. This discussion brought up the issue of paternalism versus self-determination for consumers. Paternalism and increased mechanization of care were seen as factors in the struggle by many consumers to get access to their own medical charts.

Workshop 3: Medical Statistics and the Health Care Consumer or How Not to be Snowed by the Numbers

Moderator: Louis R. Gary
Professor of Urban Planning
Hunter College Graduate Department of Urban Planning
New York, N.Y.

Panelists: Geraldine Alpert, Ph.D.
Coordinator for Data and Special Studies
Health Systems Agency of New York City

Donna Ganzer Yedvab, M.B.A.
Statistical Consultant
New York, N.Y.

A presentation by Donna Yedvab familiarized the audience with a few basic statistical concepts, such as the standard ways of expressing statistical "typicalness." Her intent was to show the variety of interpretations of the same data which can be communicated depending upon the statistical technique used. The many and varying factors that influence such common indicators of hospital use such as "length of stay" or hospital "occupancy rate" were also brought out as examples of the difficulty of relying on unexamined statistics for a single reliable meaning.

"Incidence" and "prevalence" of disease were also explained to illustrate problems in interpreting these common statistical expressions of health status. Consumers were given critical questions which must be asked in evaluating the accuracy of surveys whose purpose is to assess need for services.

Geraldine Alpert focused her presentation around two principal questions: "How are data to be used?" and "What are the problems with the data which are available to us?" She began with the caveat that data are not "a decision-making apparatus for social changes." Data are only supplemental tools that we employ to further inform ourselves. She stressed that consumers often have knowledge of the community that has not been reflected in the data. Therefore, consumer input is invaluable in making health policy.

Dr. Alpert explained the most common and readily available measures of health status: morbidity and mortality statistics. Causes for skepticism when relying on these indicators include unreliable reports of causes of death and the artifacts of increased or decreased reporting. Problems of doing accurate population-based planning were also outlined. Given the difficulties of predicting population migrations and changes in medical practice, among other factors, population-based planning may not predict accurately how many and what kinds of services will be needed in years to come.

Workshop 4: Untangling the Web of Decision Making—What Role Do (Should) Consumers Play?

Moderator: Anthony Mangiaracina
Vice-President
W. R. Grace and Co.
New York, N.Y.

Panelists: Marshall England
Executive Committee
Health Systems Agency of New York City

Bruce Mansdorf, M.P.A.
Deputy Director
New York State Health Planning and Development Agency
Albany, N.Y.

David W. Smith, J.D.
Executive Committee

Health Systems Agency of New York City
Judy Wessler
Consumer Member
Health Systems Agency of New York City

Panel presentations and the question-and-answer session in this workshop centered on effective consumer involvement in health care, especially in the health planning process. Possibilities and drawbacks were cited. Mr. Smith presented a history of consumer involvement in health planning and a brief explanation of the mandated role for consumers in the present legislation (P.L. 93–641). Although the legislation was itself a breakthrough for consumers, he expressed the view that only hard work would bring consumers into a truly influential position.

Mr. Mansdorf spoke to the issue of the relative power of the local HSAs in comparison with the state agency. He maintained that local consumers could not act responsibly as planners without an incentive to contain the total costs of health care in their service area. Putting a cap on total regional capital expenditures would be one way of inducing local planning bodies to plan in a fiscally responsible manner.

Panelists Smith and Wessler touched on the relationship (or lack of it) between consumers on the local level and those on the State Health Coordinating Council (SHCC). Ms. Wessler expressed the view that SHCC and HSA Executive Committee policy tended to be set by staff rather than members. In addition, she felt that the New York SHCC was influenced unduly by provider interests. There was discussion over the degree to which HSA and DHEW were responsible for educating and informing health consumers. Mr. England and Ms. Wessler proposed that a consumer union or consumer network was indispensable for focusing the impact of consumer interests on the system.

Part II

THE IMPACT OF MEDICAL TECHNOLOGY ON SICKNESS AND DEATH

The overall theme in this conference was linked to the assessment of medical technology from safety and efficacy viewpoints. These are major considerations for consumers to ponder when decisions have to be made. Obviously, if technological innovations can reduce mortality and mobidity, then the other values that people hold come into play. Does it cost too much? Will only a few people will be helped? Aren't other alternatives available? Questions of this nature enter the field and hold the attention of the decision makers. In a nation where huge sums are spent on "get well" cards, people do not always place a high value on community health care measures. Consumer and provider values about health care and related areas color evaluations regarding the impact of medical technology on the status of the health of the citizenry.

Is it only coincidental that the reduction in sickness and death occurred during the same time period that an avalanche of medical technology arrived on the health care scene? Positive and negative responses abound. Positions held may reflect individual biases such as your job, experience with medical technology, professional affiliations, mechanical appitude, education, social consciousness, or many other variables. Nevertheless, it should also be noted that many of the death and illness rates were already on a downward slide before the discovery and application of new medical technology. In addition, at the time of the downward trend, the general level of living in nutrition, environmental sanitation, and housing was improving. Was this another coincidence or a related causal effect?

Currently, divergent opinions about the impact of medical technology on health care appear to be gathering at the ends of the spectrum. Ivan Illich, in his book *Medical Nemesis,* [1] plays out the theme that modern medicine has reached the stage where it is itself a major threat to our health. *The Case for American Medicine,* [2] a book by Harry Schwartz, focuses upon the positive aspects of the health care system and its accomplishments. These two books are illustrative of the positions held at the ends of the continuum. Mass media, however, are focusing on the negative pole. This has made it fashionable to denigrate medical technology today. Consumers should be prepared to withhold a decision until they get all the information and not jump to a conclusion based on a newspaper story that could be taken out of context, or some other source of information that may not be giving all the facts.

In discussing the impact of drug technology on health care in the late 1800s, Dr. Oliver Wendell Holmes[3] has been quoted as saying, "I firmly believe that if the whole of the materia medica as now used could be sunk to the bottom of the sea, it would be all the better for mankind—and all the worse for the fishes." Many consumers express similar sentiments about devices and other sophisticated medical advances.

David Banta opened this second conference by relating the impact of modern technology upon the major causes of death in this country: heart disease, cancer, and stroke. Initially, Banta defined technology and health, and explored the value that we put on health. His said that there are limited resources available and limited benefits from the application of modern technology to heart disease, cancer and stroke victims. Consideration was urged for expending monies on prevention, care for the ill, and basic research on the causes of disease.

In commenting on the efficacy of clinical medical technology, Banta supported the view that improved nutrition and standards of living may have had a greater impact than technology on health status. Today, chronic diseases are our major problem as compared to 1900 when infectious diseases were predominant. Banta reviewed heart disease, cancer, and stroke in this context to lead to the plea for more research on the causes of disease. Using the example of breast cancer, Banta talked about prevention, the use of mammography, surgery, and the outcome on the health of women. His conclusion was that there are too many variables to put forth a definitive yes or no as to the applicability of technology. Again, Banta argued for a reallocation of funds to pursue investigation rather than expenditures on questionable procedures.

Banta concluded, "But it seems to me that our society is being shortsighted. Because of our faith in modern medicine, we are investing in a technological fix rather than in long-term research or prevention." His last sentence stated, "So the truth is, we just do not know the value of medical care and its technology."

As a counterbalance to Banta's position, Buxbaum related the successful use of medical technology to combat lead poisoning, calling it a technical fix for a human problem. As a case study, the facts and details about the lead poisoning situation in New York City presented a vivid picture of a definite problem. Alternative courses of action were evaluated and a choice made to use systematic screening to discover lead poisoning in children prior to actual illness. Technologic tools needed for this program were specified including a reliable laboratory test, a screening mechanism, a method of assaying lead content of paint and plaster, and an effective environmental abatement procedure. A special note was made about the introduction of microscreening techniques as well as each of the other technologies required to undertake this health care activity. In his evaluation, Buxbaum specified the positive aspects of the application of technology to a difficult public health problem. In closing, Buxbaum said that the problem of lead poisoning demands more, not less technology; more, not less innovation; and certainly more, not less effort.

The effect of health planning upon sickness and death was discussed by Fiori. She contended that improvement in the health status of people should be the central purpose and end result of health planning. The overwhelming impact of the emphasis on cost containment may, however, be working in opposition to that health planning goal. To put the health planning efforts into perspective, Fiori reviewed the current situation relative to construction of facilities, health insurance, professional specialization, primary care services, the role of influential persons in the health care system, technical and political contributions, and community life problems. Community based health planning was discussed noting the surge of consumer participation in the early 1960s and continuing into the current legislation, P.L. 93–641. With the brief historical review as a base, Fiori identified the following planning issues:

A lack of clarification of the consumer's role in health planning

An absence of adequate consumer orientation and training

Limitations in the support for consumer activities by the staff of health planning agencies

Timing and location of health planning agency activities as barriers to the involvement of consumers

Fiori noted that consumers have made significant contributions to health planning. From her vantage point, Fiori feels that consumers are ready, willing, and able to meet the challenges.

Afternoon workshops during this second conference emphasized the relationship between current medical technology applications and their impact on sickness and death. Discussions covered the use of CAT scanners; an out-of-hospital childbearing center; methods and techniques used for the prevention, detection, and treatment of breast cancer; and emergency medical services. Actual HSA Project Reviews of proposals for a CAT scanner and childbearing center were reenacted while the breast cancer and emergency medical services workshops were combinations of informative presentations and question-and-answer discussions.

Participants in the simulation of the HSA review of a CAT scanner proposal were the same people who had been involved in the real life review. This reenactment provoked typical questions to be asked by consumers sitting on review boards and by hospital staff prior to submission. An executive of the voluntary nonprofit hospital submitting the proposal defended the application. Afterwards the actual minutes of the HSA executive committee meeting were read to the audience. Members of the audience questioned the review committee panel members. The possibility of periodically reevaluating the utilization and cost effectiveness of the scanning was raised by the audience as an issue not considered at that time. Areas of concern noted by consumers related to the safety and effectiveness of CAT scanners and to the geographic distribution of the devices. Participants asked why New York City had as many scanners as Sweden and England combined. Related to the issue of need was the question of hospitals wanting CAT scanners to increase their status in the medical community.

Another workshop considered health planning, Medicaid, and *who's-at risk-for-what* aiming to identify the various interested parties. Panel members simulated the HSA review of an out-of-hospital childbearing center. Again, the actual participants were involved in the reenactment of the Maternity Center Association's 1977 application. HSA staff summaries were read and the politics of alternative versus traditional health care interests were noted during the review process. Evaluations had to be made about the risk of this innovative way of providing maternity care, especially in regard to the provision of back-up hospital services. The review panel responded to questions by audience members on birthing practices, payment methods, and data collection. A major issue raised in this workshop revolved about the role of the HSA in encouraging alternative ways of delivering health care services. Difficulties cited by HSA representatives included a lack of professional agreement on critical questions, the defensiveness of professionals and institutions when faced with consumer defections, and the needs of the consumer for low cost primary care.

Prevention, detection, and treatment of breast cancer were covered in another workshop where panelists presented information on a controversial subject. One medical expert claimed that the recent "commotion" over radiation risks from mammography was based on highly speculative evidence. While another medical expert conceded that the issue of surgery remains confusing, still another deplored the idea that women were being told that a radical mastectomy was unnecessary. A representative of a woman's health education and consumer advocacy organization disagreed with the experts on a number of points. She stated that the current self-critical attitudes and more cautious approaches of many professionals would never have come about without the prodding of the women's health care consumer movement.

Is an emergency medical service, with its sophisticated data systems, its expensive new ambulances, and highly trained personnel cost-effective? This question opened up a workshop that considered how much technology was needed for an effective emergency medical system. Historical background on the concept of "bringing the hospital to the patient" was presented by a panel member. It was noted that self-care health education for consumers could reduce the costs of emergency services by reducing unnecessary utilization. Despite the sophisticated equipment used in emergency situations, it was stated that major costs were for personnel. There was mixed data on the performance of emergency services in saving lives. Questions were raised whether mortality reduction ought to be the only criterion for the effectiveness of emergency services. Competitiveness among ambulance services was discussed and consumers stated a desire that priorities be given to burn patients, to poisoning cases, and to infants in distress. Many participants noted that while emergency medical service may be helpful, the fact that the patient's terrible living conditions remain unchanged can easily undo the positive effects of the care.

In conclusion, workshop participants spoke about the various perceptions of emergency situations and the question arose, "What is the true emergency?" No single definitive answer emerged.

REFERENCES

1. Illich, I. *Medical nemesis. The expropriation of health.* New York: Pantheon Books, 1976.
2. Schwartz, H. *The case for American medicine.* New York: David McKay Co., 1972.
3. Strauss, M. B. (ed.) *Familiar medical quotations.* Boston, Ma.: Little, Brown & Co., 1968 p. 124.

Chapter 6

MAJOR DISEASES OF MODERN AMERICA: WHAT DIFFERENCE HAS MODERN TECHNOLOGY REALLY MADE?

David Banta

This is a very broad topic and I want to look at it in a very broad context. We are faced with limited resources. When we spend on one policy or program, another suffers. I would submit that we are losing worthwhile opportunities to prevent disease and to promote health by our growing investment in the diagnosis and treatment of heart disease, cancer, and stroke. There is limited benefit from the use of these technologies. There are other important activities in the health area that we may be underfunding, especially prevention, care for the ill, and research on the causes of disease.

TECHNOLOGY AND HEALTH DEFINITIONS

What is technology?I favor a broad definition of the term. At the Office of Technology Assessment, we use the term medical technology to mean the drugs, equipment, and procedures used by health care professionals in delivering medical care to individuals and the systems within which such care is delivered. This is consistent with the dictionary definition of the word technology: "applied science."

It is also important to define health. I would choose a broad definition, emphasizing the physical, psychological, and social functioning of the individual. But our statistics, research programs, and medical care systems focus almost entirely on the physical, especially mortality. Avoiding mortality is of course a worthwhile goal, but it is also important to foster improved functioning, both physical and psychological. We set our priorities by what are the greatest causes of mortality. Tables 6–1 through 6–3 compare the leading problems in the United States by mortality, activity limitation, and hospital stays. For example, diseases of the musculoskeletal system such as arthritis are much more important in limiting activity than respiratory diseases or cancer (neoplasms). Only recently have we begun to consider other aspects of health besides physical status. This makes it hard to evaluate technology fully. Existing evaluations are almost entirely in terms of mortality.

Table 6–1 Numbers of Deaths from 10 Leading Causes, United States, 1976

Cause	Deaths
Heart disease	723,878
Cancer	377,312
Stroke	188,623
Accidents	100,761
Influenza and pneumonia	61,866
Diabetes mellitus	34,508
Cirrhosis of liver	31,453
Arteriosclerosis	29,366
Suicide	26,832
Early infancy (birth injuries, newborn infections, immaturity, ill-defined diseases, etc.)	24,809

Source: USDHEW, National Center for Health Statistics. *Facts of life and death.* Pub. No. (PHS) 79–1222. November, 1978, p. 31.

Table 6-2 Number of Persons with Limitation of Activity by Selected Chronic Conditions, United States, 1974

Heart conditions	4,753,000
Arthritis and rheumatism	4,396,000
Back or spine impairments (except paralysis)	2,051,000
Hypertension without heart involvement	1,976,000
Lower extremities and hips impaired (except paralysis)	1,889,000
Visual impairments	1,724,000
Other musculoskeletal disorders	1,718,000
Mental and nervous conditions	1,504,000
Diabetes	1,448,000
Asthma, with or without hay fever	1,434,000
Neoplasms	633,000

Data are based on household interviews of the civilian noninstitutionalized population

Source: USDHEW, National Center for Health Statistics. *Facts of life and death.* Pub. No. (PHS) 79-1222. November, 1978, p. 13.

Table 6-3 Discharges from Nonfederal Short-Stay Hospitals per 1,000 Population by First Listed Diagnosis, United States, 1974

Heart disease	20.8
Digestive system diseases	19.9
Pregnancy, childbirth complications	19.3
Accidents, poisonings	16.5
Genitourinary system	16.4
Respiratory system	15.8
Neoplasms, malignant and benign	10.9
Musculoskeletal system	8.2
Nervous system and sense organs	6.6
Mental disorders	6.5

Data are based on a sample of hospital records
Rates are based on the civilian noninstitutionalized population.

Source: USDHEW, Health Resources Administration. *Health United States 1976-1977* Pub. No. (HRA) 77-1232 1977, p. 284.

VALUE OF HEALTH

Another question is the monetary value that we put on health. The criminal justice system is clearly underfunded, but it seems likely that we could provide better justice with a larger investment. We have decided not to do that. Within the health area, we essentially put a value on health, and even on life itself, with our policy decisions. But we usually lack the courage to face that fact and to try to make rational decisions. In this situation of limited resources and multiple goals, I would argue that it is essential to see that we spend our money wisely.

EFFICACY OF HEALTH CARE

Now let me turn to the efficacy of health care and why I say that clinical medical technology is of limited value. When I use the word "efficacy" I mean simply the benefit to the individual from use of a given technology.

I will present my argument from an historical perspective. In 1850, the death rate from tuberculosis (when tuberculosis was the greatest cause of death in the U.S. population) was about 450 per 100,000 population. It then fell progressively, to 250 per 100,000 in 1890, to 115 per 100,000 in 1920, and to 36 per 100,000 in 1938. Yet, there was no specific therapy for tuberculosis until after 1938. Undoubtedly, general measures such as patient isolation had some impact before 1938. Specific therapy for tuberculosis after 1938 brought the death rate even lower. Yet, why did the bulk of the fall occur without specific measures?

McKeown,[1] working in England, studied this question by examining general death rates over a period of 140 years. He observed that death rates began falling in England about 1840. The public health revolution, however, did not begin until about 1870, and had its greatest effect after 1890. After examining all of the evidence, McKeown concluded that it was the improved nutrition and standards of living resulting from the industrial revolution that had the greatest single influence.

On the other hand, the contribution of clinical medicine to falling death rates seems to be small. Antibiotics certainly made some difference, as did modern surgery. Birth planning, with prenatal care, urging more time between children and maternal nutrition, has certainly made a difference. There are not many clear-cut examples that can be cited. Life expectancy for adults over the age of 65 has risen only 3 years since 1900. Changes in death rates and the increase in life expectancy occurred largely because of the reduction in the death rate from infectious disease in infants and young children.

Thus, my interpretation of this evidence is that there have been three historical periods:

1. Dramatically falling death rates resulted from improvements in the general environment, especially from increased standards of living and improved nutrition.
2. Further improvements from modern public health also had considerable impact through such measures as safe water supplies and immunization.
3. Clinical medicine and its technology had some impact, but a much smaller one than the first two factors. This is not to minimize the importance of medical technology, but to put it in perspective.

This points out that environmental and public health measures are likely to have had the greatest impact on health. I believe that this emphasis will continue to be true in the future. Indeed, in an era when we are making the physical environment more and more unsafe, these factors may be more important than we yet recognize.

Changing Disease Patterns

In 1900, infectious diseases were predominant; today chronic diseases are now a major problem. Figure 6–1 shows how the pattern has changed. Heart diseases, in 1900, accounted for less than 10 percent of deaths in the United States. By 1967, heart disease accounted for about 40 percent and the figure has now risen to more than 50 percent; stroke accounted for about 7 percent of deaths in 1900 and now accounts for more than 10 percent; cancer accounted for less than 5 percent of deaths in 1900, but now accounts for about 20 percent.

Again, death is not the only outcome of ill-health. These

Figure 6-1 Percentage of All Deaths by Specified Cause of Death, U.S., 1900 and 1967.

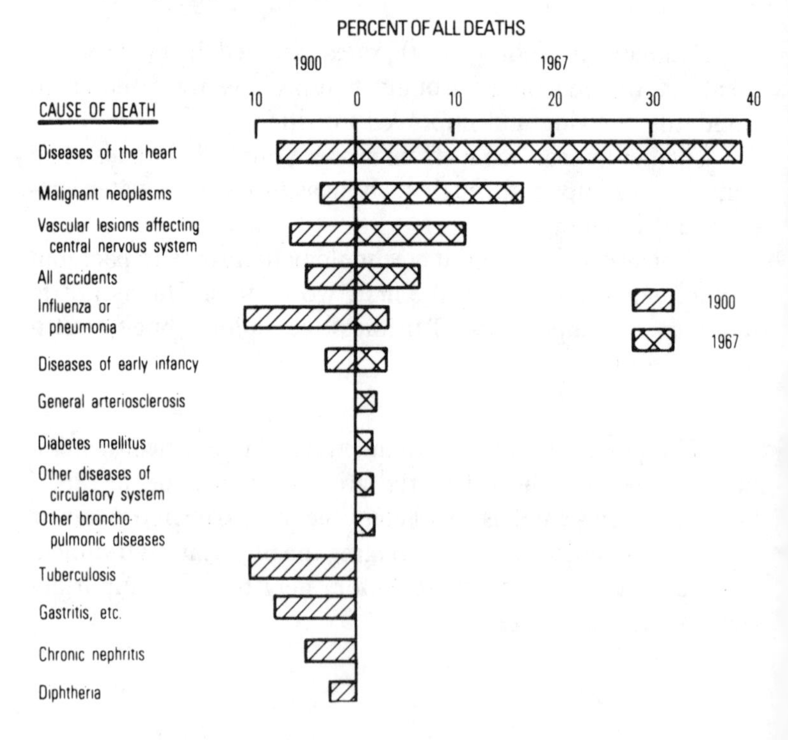

patterns would be quite different if we looked at morbidity or limitations of activity. It seems to me that we need to reorient our system to provide health care, to include attention to psychological and social functioning. This probably will not happen until we recognize the limitations of the technologic approach and change our priorities.

It is clear, however, that heart disease, cancer, and stroke are important problems. When adjusted for age (a statistical technique that takes into account that the population is older now on the average than it was in the past), the death rate has been dropping since about 1950, as seen in Table 6–4. In 1950, the age-adjusted death rate was 841 per 100,000 population and fell to about 627 per 100,000 by 1976. Table 6–1 also shows that the age-adjusted death rate for major cardiovascular diseases has been dropping since 1950 while the rate for malignant neoplasms (cancer) rose slightly over the same period.

Table 6–5 breaks down the age-adjusted death rate for major cardiovascular diseases. The bulk of the disease is "ischemic heart disease," what we ordinarily think of as heart attacks and coronary artery disease. Even after age-adjustment, those diseases actually rose until 1968 and have fallen since then; now there are about 192 per 100,000 population. On the other hand, hypertensive heart disease was a much more important cause of death in 1950 than it is now—the death rate has fallen from about 56 per 100,000 in 1950 to only about 4.8 in 1976. And the death rate from cerebrovascular diseases, or stroke, has fallen from about 89 per 100,000 in 1950 to about 51 per 100,000 in 1976.

Overall, the rate of death from cancer after age-adjustment has risen slightly since 1950. A sex breakdown of those rates indicates that cancer in males has increased considerably over the last 25 years, while the death rate from cancer in females has stayed about the same. The most dramatic change, however, is the striking increase in deaths from lung cancer in males, due, of course, almost entirely to cigarette smoking (Fig. 6–2). Stomach cancer deaths have decreased markedly in both sexes, as have uterine cancer deaths in women. We can see the

Table 6–4 Age-Adjusted Death Rates for Selected Causes: United States, 1950–1976
[Rates per 100,000 population.]

Year	*All causes* (1)	*Malignant neoplasms, including neoplasms of lymphatic and hematopoietic tissues*[1] (2)	*Major cardiovascular diseases*[2] (3)	*All other diseases*[3] (4)	*Accidents, poisonings, and violence*[4] (5)
1976[5]	627.5	132.3	284.4	143.6	67.2
1975[5]	638.3	130.9	291.4	145.8	70.2
1974[5]	666.2	131.8	310.8	152.1	71.5
1973[5]	692.9	130.7	326.9	158.7	76.6
1972[5, 6]	701.8	130.7	333.8	160.4	76.9
1971[5]	699.9	129.7	334.8	159.1	76.3
1970[5]	714.3	129.9	340.1	166.9	77.4
1969	728.5	128.9	350.4	171.5	77.7
1968	743.8	129.2	361.8	176.3	76.5
1967	725.6	128.1	362.6	161.3	73.6
1966	742.2	127.5	374.0	167.4	73.3
1965	739.0	127.0	374.2	166.9	70.9
1964	739.4	125.9	376.6	168.2	68.7
1963	756.9	126.1	388.6	174.6	67.6
1962	745.5	125.2	386.1	168.1	66.1
1961	735.6	125.2	381.6	165.0	63.8
1960	760.9	125.8	393.5	175.9	65.7

1959	750.9	124.5	391.2	169.8	65.4
1958	764.6	124.6	400.2	174.6	65.2
1957	776.3	126.4	403.1	178.9	67.9
1956	763.3	126.3	396.5	171.4	69.1
1955	764.6	125.8	396.1	173.6	69.1
1954	763.2	125.8	392.5	176.8	68.1
1953	804.7	125.9	412.7	193.9	72.2
1952	815.8	125.7	414.5	201.7	73.9
1951	829.1	124.3	420.1	210.3	74.4
1950[7]	841.5	125.4	425.6	216.6	73.9

[1] For 1958–1976 rates are based on deaths assigned to category numbers 140–209 of the *Eighth Revision of the International Classification of Diseases, Adapted for Use in the United States*, adopted in 1965; for 1950–1967 rates are based on deaths assigned to category numbers 140–205 of the Sixth and Seventh Revisions adopted, respectively, in 1948 and 1955.

[2] For 1958–1976 rates are based on deaths assigned to category numbers 390–448 of the *Eighth Revision of the International Classification of Diseases, Adapted for Use in the United States*, adopted in 1965; for 1950–1967 rates are based on deaths assigned to category numbers 330–334, 400–468 of the Sixth and Seventh Revisions adopted, respectively, in 1948 and 1955.

[3] Residual: Column (1) less columns (2), (3), and (5).

[4] For 1968–1976 rates are based on deaths assigned to category numbers E800–E999 of the *Eighth Revision of the International Classification of Diseases, Adapted for Use in the United States*, adopted in 1965; for 1950–1967 rates are based on deaths assigned to category numbers E800–E964, E970–E985 of the Sixth and Seventh Revisions adopted, respectively, in 1948 and 1955. Data for 1950–1967 exclude injury resulting from operations of war (ICD Nos. E965, E990–E999). This does not appreciably destroy comparability; for the greatest frequency of deaths in the United States from such injuries was 74 for 1966. These deaths for operations of war are included in all other diseases for the years 1950–1967.

[5] Excludes deaths of nonresidents of the United States.

[6] Based on a 50-percent sample of deaths.

[7] Based on enumerated population adjusted for age bias in the population of races other than white.

Source: Division of Vital Statistics, National Center for Health Statistics, 1977.

Table 6–5 Age-Adjusted Death Rates for Major Cardiovascular Diseases and Components: United States, 1950–1976

[Rates per 100,000 population]

Year	*Total*[1]	*Active rheumatic fever and chronic rheumatic heart disease*[2]	*Hypertensive heart disease with or without renal disease; and hypertension*[3]	*Ischemic heart disease*[4]	*Cerebrovascular diseases*[5]	*Other major cardiovascular diseases (residual)*
1976[6]	284.4	4.7	4.8	191.6	51.4	31.9
1975[6]	291.4	4.8	5.1	196.1	54.5	30.9
1974[6]	310.8	5.1	5.7	207.7	59.9	32.4
1973[6]	326.9	5.4	6.3	218.9	63.7	32.6
1972[6, 7]	333.8	5.7	6.9	223.9	65.0	32.3
1971[6]	334.8	6.0	7.2	225.1	65.2	31.3
1970[6]	340.1	6.3	7.8	228.1	66.3	31.6
1969	350.4	6.6	8.5	234.7	68.3	32.3
1968	361.8	7.2	9.4	241.6	71.3	32.3
1967	362.6	6.5	22.2	211.8	69.7	52.4
1966	374.0	7.0	24.3	216.6	72.3	53.8
1965	374.2	7.4	25.2	215.8	72.7	53.1
1964	376.6	7.7	26.9	215.4	73.6	53.0
1963	388.6	8.2	29.1	220.3	76.4	54.6
1962	386.1	8.9	30.1	216.9	76.6	53.6
1961	381.6	9.1	31.1	211.4	76.7	53.3
1960	393.5	9.6	33.7	214.6	79.7	55.9

1959	391.1	9.7	35.4	210.4	80.7	54.9
1958	400.2	10.1	39.3	210.4	83.0	57.4
1957	403.1	11.1	38.5	211.2	84.2	58.1
1956	396.5	11.2	39.4	205.1	82.3	58.5
1955	396.1	11.2	41.4	200.0	83.0	60.5
1954	392.5	11.4	43.5	193.4	83.0	61.2
1953	412.7	12.5	48.7	196.1	86.9	68.5
1952	414.6	12.9	51.7	190.2	87.8	72.0
1951	420.2	13.3	54.3	187.0	89.0	76.6
1950[8]	425.6	14.0	56.0	185.2	88.8	81.6

[1] For 1968–1976 rates are based on deaths assigned to category numbers 390–448 of the *Eighth Revision of the International Classification of Diseases, Adapted for Use in the United States*, adopted in 1965; for 1950–1967 rates are based on deaths assigned to category numbers 330–334, 440–468 of the Sixth and Seventh Revisions adopted, respectively, in 1948 and 1955.

[2] For 1968–1976 rates are based on deaths assigned to category numbers 390–398 of the *Eighth Revision of the International Classification of Diseases, Adapted for Use in the United States*, adopted in 1965; for 1950–1967 rates are based on deaths assigned to category numbers 400–402, 410–416 of the Sixth and Seventh Revisions adopted, respectively, in 1948 and 1955.

[3] For 1968–1976 rates are based on deaths assigned to category numbers 400–404 of the *Eighth Revision of the International Classification of Diseases, Adapted for Use in the United States*, adopted in 1965; for 1950–1967 rates are based on deaths assigned to category numbers 440–447 of the Sixth and Seventh Revisions adopted, respectively, in 1948 and 1955.

[4] For 1968–1976 rates are based on deaths assigned to category numbers 410–413 of the *Eighth Revision of the International Classification of Diseases, Adapted for Use in the United States*, adopted in 1965; for 1950–1967 rates are based on deaths assigned to category number 420 of the Sixth and Seventh Revisions adopted, respectively, in 1948 and 1955.

[5] For 1968–1976 rates are based on deaths assigned to category numbers 430–438 of the *Eighth Revision of the International Classification of Diseases, Adapted for Use in the United States*, adopted in 1965; for 1950–1967 rates are based on deaths assigned to category numbers 330–334 of the Sixth and Seventh Revisions adopted, respectively, in 1948 and 1955.

[6] Excludes deaths of nonresidents of the United States.

[7] Based on a 50-percent sample of deaths.

[8] Based on enumerated population adjusted for age bias in the population of races other than white.

Source: Division of Vital Statistics, National Center for Health Statistics, 1977.

Figure 6–2 Time Trends in Cancer Mortality Rates, by Site and Sex, U.S., 1930–1970.

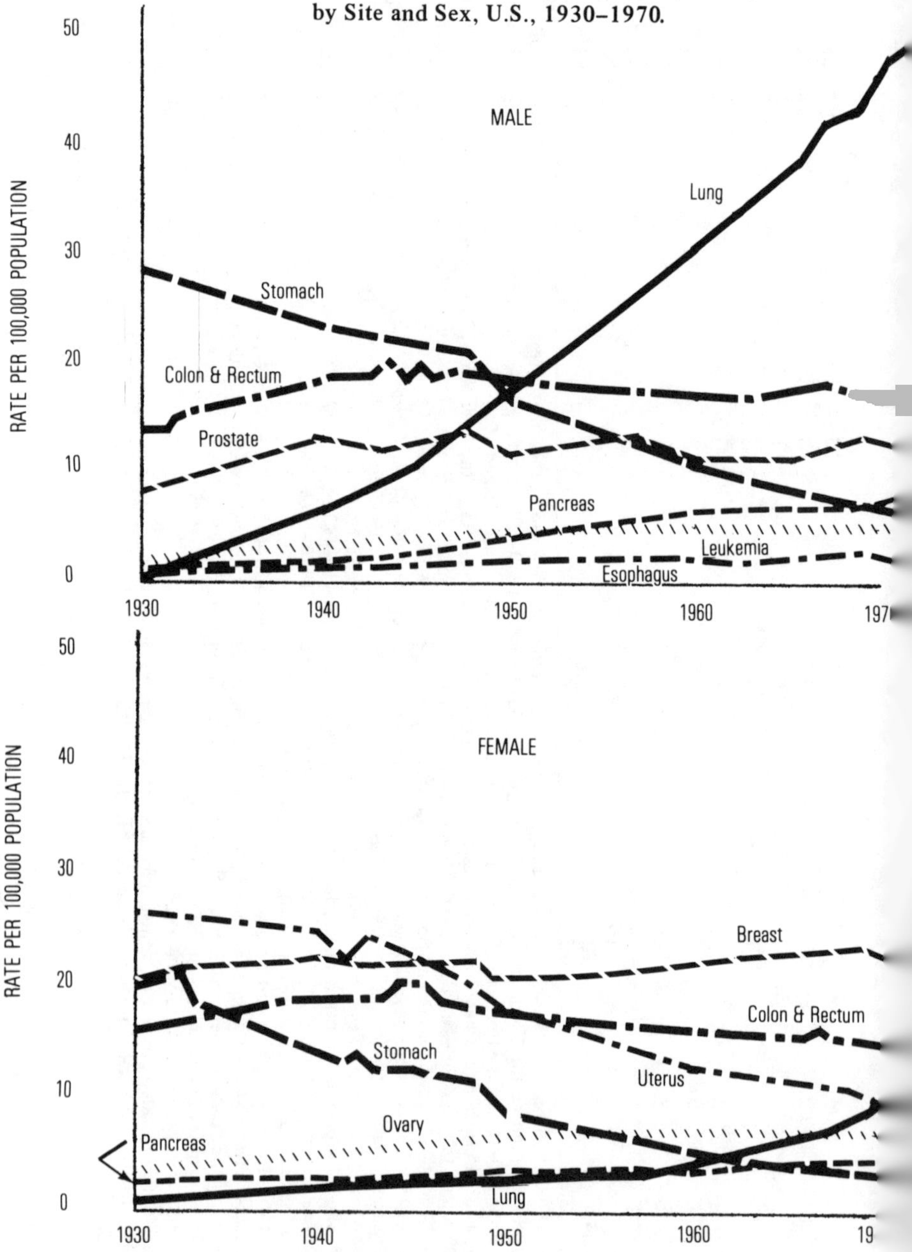

Source: U.S. DHEW, NIH, *Cancer Rates and Risks*, 1974.

beginning of a steep rise in lung cancer death rates in women, attributable to increased smoking. Most cancer deaths are now from cancer of the lung, prostate, and colon and rectum in men, and breast, colon and rectum and cervix in women.

First, why have the heart disease death rate and the stroke death rate fallen? Basically, we do not know. We have the knowledge to prevent much of the burden of these diseases. We know that if people stop smoking, exercise, watch their diet, and have effective treatment for hypertension, heart disease deaths can be prevented. But with the exception of hypertension, none of these factors has changed enough over the past 25 years to explain a falling death rate. Treatment for hypertension began in the 1950s and this probably made a major contribution. The same could be said for stroke deaths, which are often related to high blood pressure. As for treatment technology, the evidence for any impact from emergency care, coronary care units, and so forth is not very convincing. Nevertheless, there probably has been some impact from such efforts.

We know that smoking in males explains a great part of the rising cancer death rate. We are beginning to see a rapid rise in death rates from lung cancer in women because of changing smoking habits. Otherwise, we know from epidemiological studies that environment, broadly defined to include diet and cigarette smoking, causes 80 to 90 percent of cancers. However, that does not mean that we have the specific knowledge necessary to make prevention of those cancers possible. We could perhaps prevent 40 percent or so of cancers and cancer deaths now with available knowledge. The fact that half or more of those would be cancers due to smoking indicates how limited our knowledge is. This points out the need for more research on the causes of disease.

TECHNOLOGY AND MAJOR ILLNESS

What about the usefulness of the technologies applied to these three major conditions? It is difficult to generalize—there are too many specific disease conditions and too many technologies in use. Furthermore, the evaluations that have been done have focused on the easy outcome to measure, mortality. I can say that except for the clear-cut example of the treatment of hypertension and treatment for Hodgkin's disease, a form of cancer, there have not been too many dramatic successes.

Let me illustrate some of the complexities by discussing some aspects of one disease and its prevention and treatment. During the past 25 years, breast cancer, the most common cause of cancer death in women, has increased slightly but the survival has only improved slightly. Thus, the death rate has stayed about the same, a little more than 20 per 100,000 per year. Most women with breast cancer (62 percent) are treated with surgery. Three-year survival was 63 percent in 1950 and has risen to 72 percent by the late 1960s and early 1970s. Of course this is not a dramatic change.

We do not know enough about prevention. We know from epidemiological studies that breast cancer is higher in white women, that it runs in families, that it is higher in single women and lower in women with early childbearing, that it is higher in the upper socioeconomic classes, and that it is higher in women with a high fat intake in their diets. These associations are obviously not of too much help in preventing the disease. Because of this, the idea of screening to find breast cancer early developed. It is known that if cancer is found early in its development, it can quite often be treated effectively, and perhaps even cured. Mammography, a special x-ray of the breast, has been used for this purpose, in conjunction with physician examination and self-examination. Mammography was developed in the 1930s and it still being evaluated. At first, mammography was shown to be an effective tool for the diagnosis of breast cancer. Then, the idea developed to use it as part of periodic screening programs. This idea was tested in a controlled clinical trial carried out in the Health Insurance Plan of Greater New York (HIP) during the mid-1960s. In the study, 60,000 women were randomly assigned to a study or control group. The study group was screened periodically for breast cancer. At the end of 7 years, there were 70 deaths in the study group and 108 in the control group. This is a statistically significant difference. This finding led the American Cancer Society and the National Institutes of Health to start a breast cancer demonstration project. So far that project has enrolled more than 270,000 women. By 1975, however, questions were being raised about the x-ray exposure women had from mammography. Studies had been completed showing the x-ray to the breast causes cancer itself. So the question became how to balance the benefits and risks. Data from the HIP study was analyzed again, and it was recognized that its results showed no benefit in women under the age of 50. Therefore, the National Institutes of Health recommended screening by mammography only for women over the age of 50 or with particular risk factors. Many radiologists disagreed with this decision. These doctors argued that the technology of mammography had improved greatly in the last 10 years, that the radiation dose was lower, and that many women under the age of 50 with early breast cancer had been found with mammography. This controversy continues. The HIP study is the only well-designed study of this subject. Despite its findings, widespread screening of women under the age of 50 continues.

Turning to therapy, radical mastectomy is often considered the standard treatment for breast cancer. Radical mastectomy is the removal of the breast and surrounding tissues by surgery in an attempt to get rid of all of the cancer. It is a mutilating and traumatic procedure. There have been questions about its benefits for years. In recent years almost 100,000 operations have been done every year. In 1971, the National Institutes of Health started a controlled clinical trial of breast cancer treatment, including radical mastectomy. Preliminary results show radical mastectomy to be no better than simple mastectomy in terms of survival. Although these results are preliminary, they certainly raise questions about the usefulness of radical mastectomy. They also raise questions about why the procedure was not evaluated earlier.

These results cause one to question many other commonly

used technologies, especially operative procedures. If we spend money on such expensive surgery, obviously we cannot spend it on research or prevention or on other worthwhile programs. This seems a particular shame when the procedure is questionable or of no benefit. I am often asked if this is a real problem. The answer is yes. In the budget of the Department of Health, Education and Welfare, the rapidly rising expenditures for the Medicare and Medicaid programs are squeezing the other budgets of the Department, including the traditional prevention programs.

Summary

In summary, I cannot make a simple statement about technology in heart disease, cancer, and stroke. Each problem and patient have to be thought of individually. But it seems that we are shortsighted; because of our faith in modern medicine, we are investing in a technologic fix rather than in long-term research or prevention. We are not assuring good social conditions for all our citizens. We are not assuring good nutrition. We are hardly trying to assure that everyone has the best chance to live a fulfilled life. And we are not training physicians to value prevention and to help their patients adopt healthy behavior.

Why does our medical care system behave the way it does? I believe that it is a broad societal problem: an excessive faith in technology. When we realize that much of this faith is misplaced, and that technology cannot compensate for years of destructive behavior or for the ravages of age, perhaps we will change our priorities. I would also note that many people do not choose—and probably would not choose—the dramatic technology when they are ill. Respirators, the renal dialysis machines, the electronic fetal monitors are often provided because of professional preferences, not because patients made enlightened choices. We know little about the efficacy of medical technology. As illustrated by the case of breast cancer, few studies have been done. And when studies are done, they do not necessarily modify the behavior of health care professionals and administrators. Even the studies that are done concern themselves with physical health and rarely occupy themselves with functioning or the quality of life. So the truth is, we just do not know the value of medical care and its technology.

Reference

1. McKeown, T., Record, R. G. & Turner, R. D. An interpretation of the decline of mortality in England and Wales during the twentieth century. *Population Studies.* 1975, 29, 391–422.

Chapter 7

LEAD POISONING: TECHNICAL FIX FOR A HUMAN PROBLEM

Joel N. Buxbaum

Overview

In March of 1969, Rene Dubos chaired an international symposium on childhood lead poisoning held in New York City. In summarizing the content of the two-day meeting, he closed by exclaiming:[1]

> The problem (lead poisoning) is so well defined, so neatly packaged with the causes and cures known, that if we don't eliminate this social crime our society deserves all the disasters that have been forecast for it.

Dr. Dubos was quite correct in principle. The health effects of lead were well known at this time. Fatal outcomes were unusual, but seizures and other central nervous system disorders, anemia, and kidney disease had been documented in both children and occupationally exposed adults for many years. Association between the symptoms of lead poisoning and the ingestion of lead-containing paint by children afflicted with pica (the ingestion of nonfood objects) had been documented for 40 years.

Much scattered data suggested that lead poisoning was a

major disease of New York City children. In the absence of a systematic detection program, some 143 cases of childhood lead poisoning had been noted in the city from 1950 to 1955; 27 percent of those children died. Under the leadership of Dr. H. Jacobziner,[2] 338 cases were diagnosed by the New York City Health Department in 1963. These patients were discovered only because of increased awareness of the problem among health professionals. No attempt had been made to find these children before they became ill. With Dr. Jacobziner's death, the consciousness of the prevalence and seriousness of the disease waned among the members of the medical and public health communities. Hence, in 1967 and 1968, only 4000 to 5000 blood lead determinations were performed by the N.Y.C. Health Department laboratory. Approximately 10 percent of these values were elevated and 1 percent of the cases had a fatal outcome.

A number of small screening studies were carried out in various central city communities. Resulting data suggested that the true incidence of increased lead exposure, as determined by elevated blood levels, ranged between 6 and 40 percent of the children examined. Factors that appeared to be responsible were old housing, previously painted with paints having a high lead content, and deterioration of that housing usually related to poor maintenance and children with pica. In the presence of heavily leaded paint chips, children going through the developmental stage when normal mouthing behavior occurs were also at great risk. It was estimated that there were 450,000 such dwelling units in New York City and these could have been housing 120,000 children between the ages of 1 and 6.

Alternative Actions

These were the facts as Dr. Dubos knew them. What course of action did they suggest? Clearly, it was a question of separating the child from the menace. What were the public health options? Substandard housing could not be demolished because there was already a shortage of low- and middle-income housing in the city. Since the total environment could not be deleaded, only those dwellings representing a clear and present danger could be attacked. The technology of environmental lead detection required extensive paint and plaster sampling, a procedure which the Health Department had abandoned 5 years earlier as not being cost-effective. In addition, the Health Code of New York City did not support random screening of apartments as a preventive measure prior to detection of a child with lead poisoning. Hence, selective abatement of the hazard was not practicable. A third alternative represented the application of an "after the fact" technology. Children already exposed to excessive lead would be detected by systematic screening prior to the time they became ill. This last approach was deemed most applicable in New York City.

Necessary Technologic Tools

What were the technologic tools necessary to achieve the goals stated by Dr. Dubos? These included the following:

- A reliable, acceptable method of determining excess body burden of lead
- A mechanism whereby the majority, if not all, of the children at risk could be tested
- A simple, rapid method of assaying the lead content of paint and plaster
- An effective way of environmental abatement

All of these appeared to be available in 1969, but were they really able to be used?

A standard method of blood lead determination using dithizone had been available for many years; however, the test required 5 ml of whole blood. Because of the small veins of young children, such a sample was difficult to obtain. Often, the services of a skilled physician was required to obtain blood from the large jugular vein of the neck. Many parents were unwilling to allow their children to undergo such a drastic sampling procedure. For mass screening, two alternative strategies were available. Both required the development of an analytic technique that could be performed reliably with small samples of blood, preferably a sample that could be obtained from a finger puncture.

Atomic absorption spectroscopy had already been employed for the quantitative microanalysis of lead in other settings. Hence, after an appropriate stimulus, the laboratories of the New York City Health Department, under the perceptive leadership of Dr. Bernard Davidow, developed a method for processing small samples of blood so that they could be subjected to atomic absorption analysis.

Simultaneously, investigators working in departments of pediatrics in various parts of the country attempted to develop a technology based on earlier observations which had shown that even small amounts of lead could alter the metabolism of hemoglobin in the body's red blood cells. The altered metabolism resulted in the accumulation of substances in the blood and urine which could be measured easily. Several attempts were made to apply urine tests to pediatric screening. Although most of these proved satisfactory for adults, they proved to be unreliable when applied to 1- to 6-year-olds.

Other investigators concentrated their efforts on measuring such substances in the blood. The most successful of these scientists was Dr. Sergio Piomelli[3] of the New York University Medical School. Working in the Department of Pediatric Hematology at Bellevue Hospital, he established that one of the substances which accumulated in red blood cells in the presence of lead, free erythrocyte protoporphyrin (FEP) could be measured readily in a small amount of blood. Further, he noted that the stability of the compound was such that a drop of blood could be collected on a piece of filter paper and transported to a central laboratory that could then process large numbers of samples rapidly. Dr. Piomelli's work was a major technical breakthrough.

Additional Methods Needed

Development of microscreening techniques clearly facilitated large-scale screening. The recruitment of children and parents, however, to have their blood tested demanded the concomitant development of methodologies appropriate not only to test larger numbers of children but also to insure that those most at risk had access to testing.

Original approaches involved the application of brute force to those communities which were known to contain deteriorating housing and had a history of frequent cases of lead poisoning. Television advertising, the use of indigenous community action groups cooperating with mobile testing laboratories, increasing the awareness of Health Department personnel working in well baby clinics, and professional education resulted in a rapid increase in the number of blood lead determinations performed by the central Health Department laboratory. From the 500 to 1000 tests performed in 1968, the number leaped to 10,000 in 1969, to 85,000 in 1970, and to a peak of 124,000 in 1974.

With the increase in screening activity, the number of children found to have dangerously elevated lead levels skyrocketed. At that time, a blood lead concentration of 60 mg per dl of blood was considered to represent disease. In 1966, only 466 such cases were reported; in 1970, over 5000 children were found to have blood lead levels in the dangerous range. Children were finally being located.

What happened when the children were found? Those with high lead levels were hospitalized and treated. Technical advances requisite for therapy had already been defined at a number of institutions. Dr. Julian Chisolm[4] of the Johns Hopkins Medical School had developed a therapy protocol which minimized the previously severe side effects of therapy. Later, other groups were to successfully attempt the oral treatment of the disease with other drugs. Hence, the children could be at least partially deleaded.

ENVIRONMENTAL TECHNOLOGY

But what about the environment? Could the lead in the home or play area be identified and the environment modified so that the child would not return to the surroundings originally responsible for its conditon. This approach was both administrative and technical. The previously cancelled sampling procedure was reinstated, with multiple samples being taken from the apartments of stricken children. Assays of these samples were also facilitated by the availability of atomic absorption. Mere institution of the more rigorous sampling techniques increased the yield of positive samples from the dwellings of afflicted children from 20 percent in 1969 to 80 percent in 1971. A number of attempts were made to develop instruments that could rapidly scan an entire apartment including the intact walls. Although an instrument with such a capability was developed in the Department of Environmental Medicine at New York University Medical Center, it proved unsuitable for field work. Similar devices have been utilized in other communites, but to date none have been proven reliable in New York City.

After an apartment had been noted to be heavily leaded, new approaches were necessary to insure that a poisoned child would not become repoisoned on return home. A formal procedure was established that allowed the city's emergency repair program to provide abatement if the landlord failed to do so within a specified time. Landlords would then be billed for the costs. Various techniques of abatement were tried. The most protective appeared to be the installation of wall board to a height of four feet. Window sills and door jams (usually heavily leaded) would be scraped to bare wood and repainted or replaced. Even after 10 years of experience, it is still not clear what method of repair is most effective in preventing repoisoning.

In 1970 and 1971, when it was very evident that 20 percent of the children with elevated blood levels were neither living nor playing in homes with lead-bearing walls, a search began for other sources. An obvious fact was noted: most of the lead smelted in the world was added to gasoline as an antiknock compound. Some 100,000 tons of lead were burned each year in automobile engines in the United States.

Lead is a cumulative toxin and its effects occur no matter what the source. Therefore, it seemed reasonable to attempt to further lower the total environmental lead burden of these children by reducing or removing the lead in gasoline. City ordinances mandating the gradual removal of lead from gasoline were instituted. These ordinances would have been totally ineffective had the major automobile manufacturers not decided to build automobile engines which could run efficiently on low-lead or lead-free gasoline and to comply with the standards set by the Federal Clean Air Act of 1967.[5] Hence, a developing automotive technology allowed an administrative action to be effective and enforceable.

Evaluation

In 1978, we can look at the results of nine years of development and application of technology to a very human problem. We see successes; on the basis of 100,000 first blood specimens examined yearly, we can see a decrease in the number of children with dangerously increased body burdens of lead. In 1970, 2,469 children had blood lead levels above 55 mg per dl. In 1976, only 370 children were similarly affected. In 1977, an even smaller number had that much lead in their blood. From

1954 to 1970, there was an average of 10 lead poisoning deaths per year in New York City; since 1970, there have been but 4 such cases, the last occurring in 1974. In addition, the mean blood lead level of children between the ages of 25 and 36 months living in the city of New York has dropped between 25 and 30 percent.[6]

These are the positive aspects of the application of technology to a difficult public health problem. Are they the effect of the implementation of a technologic fix? Perhaps, but innovations in data acquisition during the 1970s allowed us to learn new facts from the old principles. It now seems clear that we can no longer be sanguine about what were formerly considered to be safe levels of lead in the blood. It can be demonstrated in the test tube that any amount of lead will inhibit certain sensitive metabolic pathways, at least one of which is readily found in brain cells.

Children with moderate blood lead levels between 40 and 50 mg per dl have been shown to have deficits in certain intellectual functions when compared with their peers who have blood lead levels below 30 mg. A group of children with hyperkinetic behavioral disorders without a known cause has been found to have a larger body burden of lead than a similar goup of children with hyperkinesis of known origin. The technology of scientific investigation and data acquistition allowed us to discover these terribly disturbing aspects of lead poisoning. We know what price the most seriously poisoned children have paid for the lead burden we have given them. We can only guess at the price that the unrecognized sufferers have paid in educational failure and social disruptiveness.

It is clear that in the past nine years New York City has attempted to heed Dr. Dubos' call to arms. No longer does the city deserve the disasters that were forecast for it. In the process, however, the problem has become more subtle and the effects more difficult to accommodate. Today, the problem of lead poisoning demands more, not less, technology; more, not less, innovation; and certainly more, not less, effort.

References

1. Dubos, R. Conference Summary at conference on Lead Poisoning in Children held at Rockefeller University, New York, N.Y., March 25–26, 1969
2. Jacobziner, H. Lead poisoning in childhood: Epidemiology, manifestations and prevention. *Clinical Pediatrics.* 1966, *5,* 277–286.
3. Piomelli, S. A micromethod for free erythroycte porphyrins: the FEP test. *Journal of Laboratory and Clinical Medicine.* 1973, 81, 932–940.
4. Chisolm, J. J. Jr. Treatment of lead poisoning. *Modern Treatment.* 1971, *8,* 593–612.
5. U.S. Congress Air Quality Act of 1967 P.L. 90–148.
6. New York City Health Services Administration. *Annual report, 1978.* page 7.

Chapter 8

HEALTH PLANNING: CAN IT AFFECT SICKNESS AND DEATH?

Florence B. Fiori

PLANNING GOALS

Improvement in the health status of people should be the central purpose and end result of health planning. This perspective is often lost in our current focus on cost containment. These two issues are not unrelated. Many individuals can attest personally to the fact that the United States is currently experiencing extremely high expenditures for health services. At the same time, health status in the United States is lower in many respects than it needs to be as evidenced by comparison data from other countries.

Health planning efforts should attempt to address the questions that this situation raises. Planners should seek more effective ways to utilize financial resources which may become increasingly scarce.

All the issues involved are not simple or easy to resolve. There are no magic answers. All of us who are engaged in health planning recognize that the field is in a very elementary stage of development. We have a long way to go if we are to achieve sound and reliable planning methods. There are probably very few final answers.

While this may sound discouraging, the nature of the work is both exciting and hopeful. These limits of knowledge are not peculiar to health planning. Many other fields face similar problems. From my point of view, we are currently in a better position than ever before to address, as a nation, our commitment to meeting the health needs of the entire population through the use of health planning as an increasingly accepted and important tool.

Goals of health planning should aim to improve health status in such a way as to minimize sickness and to prolong the inevitability of death. To meet this goal will require creativity, competence and a lot of determination. It will also require considerably better use of resources which are likely to remain the same or shrink in the face of continuing inflation. Better use of resources should be a principal result of planning.

Where Are We?

I am not nearly so concerned about how I allocate my resources when my bank account shows a hefty balance as I am when it looks like the budget is running low. At that point, I must be much more careful to ensure that income will meet expenditures and that expenditures are made for those items that will have the most benefit. That is about where we are at in terms of the health needs of people and the dollars available to meet those needs. How did we get to this point? A summary taken from the text of an educational package and based upon a document entitled "Trends in the Delivery of Health Services in the United States" may help to explain.

Construction

At the end of World War II, government funding of research stimulated medical discoveries, many of which required elaborate equipment and highly specialized personnel to put into practice. Hill-Burton monies helped finance the construction of hospitals to house the new equipment. Eventually, Medicare reimbursement of hospitals for depreciation enabled these institutions to add ever more sophisticated equipment. Government research grants accelerated the growth in the prestige and influence of medical schools and their affiliated teaching hospitals. These institutions, in turn, inspired increasing specialization among doctors and intensified interest in care requiring expensive technology.

Health Insurance

Expansion of health insurance and the inauguration of Medicare reinforced these trends in three ways:

1. Since coverage was better for impatient care than ambulatory care, an incentive was created to get needed care in a hospital whenever possible.
2. Physicians and their patients felt little constraint to economize on the type of hospital care used since insurance or Medicare paid most hospital bills.
3. With third-party insurers reimbursing hospitals for almost all costs, no matter how rapidly those costs rose, administrators had little incentive to economize and acceded to doctors' requests for the installation of new facilities and services. In effect, health insurance and Medicare removed the restraint of price competition from our health care system.

Complexity

At the same time, the growing complexity of medicine fostered specialization among doctors. Specialists, increasingly staffing community hospitals, pressured "their" hospitals to add the equipment required by their diverse specialties. This contributed to the geographic maldistribution of doctors because specialists need access to a hospital with the sophisticated equipment less likely to be found in remote rural areas. Growing specialization of doctors also meant that few in the medical world were in a position to evaluate the overall health care needs of a community or of a hospital or even of a patient.

Until recently the development of health care was guided, in good measure, by the scientific and economic interests of those who provide health care. There have been few effective mechanisms for the consumer to exercise much influence. Hospitals became the keystone of the system. It was largely the physicians, however, who determined what services were to be offered and in what institutions with what equipment. Third parties routinely paid a good portion of the bills. While some consumers were receiving excellent, and, at times, too elaborate, secondary and tertiary care in hospitals, others were crowding emergency rooms for simple primary care or were unable to get care at all.

Eventually our emphasis on top quality secondary and tertiary care pushed health care costs so high that government, health insurers, and the public grew alarmed. Government at various levels instituted rate regulation, regulations to curb capital expenditures, comprehensive health planning, and Professional Standards Review Organizations to review hospital utilization. Health Maintenance Organizations, which provide comprehensive health care for a fixed monthly fee, were promoted. Health insurers experimented with various types of cost controls. Health insurance was expanded to provide better coverage of outpatient care and thus to reduce the incentive to use expensive inpatient care unnecessarily.

PRIMARY CARE

Responding to consumer complaints about inadequate primary care (and concerned that this inadequacy was stimulating the inflation in health care costs), government has sought to put more emphasis on primary care. Federal research grants have been cut back, and this may in time lead to a slower rate of technologic change in medicine. Hill-Burton funds have been reduced, and those that remain are increasingly used for outpatient rather than inpatient facilities. Neighborhood health centers have been built with the aid of government funds. The National Health Service Corps was created in an effort to place doctors in underserved areas. This goal may also be promoted by a program of loan forgiveness for medical students who agree to practice for a time in these areas. Partly because of government encouragement, medical schools and teaching hospitals began to expand their training in "family medicine."

Increasingly sensitive to community pressures, hospitals began to reorganize their outpatient and emergency departments to provide primary care that could not be obtained elsewhere. Some hospitals sponsored neighborhood health centers. Many hospitals hired foreign medical graduates and physician assistants to alleviate physician shortages. Gaps in our health care system began to be filled by public and private programs.

Centers of Influence

Our complex health care structure is changing. Centers of influence in the system appear to be moving toward hospital administrators and government regulators. Hospitals are making some effort to coordinate their work with other institutions, and in some instances to share services or even to merge. Consumers, better educated and more affluent, are finding ways to make their voices heard through malpractice suits, pressure on legislators and regulators, and representation on hospital boards and Health Systems Agencies (HSAs).

We have a system that has grown on the basis of short-term immediate demands. These demands come most often from those who provide service rather than from those who receive it. These demands are generally made without constraints or concerns related to long-range benefits or costs.

Technical and Political Contributions

A major responsibility of the HSAs created under P.L. 93–641 (The National Health Planning and Resources Development Act) is to change this approach while preserving the strength of the current system. Both provider and consumer members of HSAs have important contributions to make. These contributions relate to two major tasks, one technical and the other political.

In some respects, the technical part of the job is the newest and the hardest part of what confronts us. Little is known about the best way to look at existing problems or to plan for their long-range resolution. We are not often certain about how to contrast the benefits of a particular health service with what it costs to provide that service. Much of the data needed for good health planning is not readily available to health planning agencies or, if available, is not subjected to rigorous study and analysis. The list of problems seems endless. But in spite of these problems, progress is occurring. From my point of view, at least some of this progress is a direct result of the more detailed law, regulations, and guidance provided by the federal government. P. L. 93–641 and the financial resources for health planning that it provides are strong evidence of increased federal commitment to the identification of health needs and to the development of appropriate resources to meet the needs.

On the political side of health planning there is more history but perhaps even larger problems. Federally sponsored health planning, in its present form and in the earlier comprehensive health planning legislation of 1966, has as a principal thrust the increased involvement of the public in decision making surrounding the identification and resolution of existing health problems. This is expected to occur through the organization and operation of representative boards and committees of health planning agencies; through the conduct of agency business in an openly public manner; and through an aggressive program of public education about health planning issues. The focus is upon organized community (i.e., political) action for health. This type of activity is not new nor is it peculiar to our particular time and place.

Community Life Problems

Rosen,[1] in his survey of community action for health establishes that "throughout human history, the major problems of health that men have faced have been concerned with community life." Evidence of organized social effort to improve the physical environment and the provision of medical care exists in abundance and preceeds the Christian era.

As nations were developed their interest was linked closely to the value of healthy and productive human resources and to the more altruistic concern of protection of the weak and the needy. National governments in various parts of the world translated this concern into the development of social policy and the provision of related services, most often prompted by occurrence of pestilence and massive outbreaks of communicable disease.

The United States, however, has lagged noticeably behind its closest social and cultural counterparts, Western Europe and Canada. Some attribute this lag to our national tendency toward free enterprise, laissez faire development, and antipathy toward government intervention. In the past, these tendencies have been countered from time to time by periods of reform and the zeal of various private reform minded groups. Efforts to solve health problems have generally been initiated at the local level. As problems grew in scope and intensity, the states and federal government became involved.

In the 1910 to 1920 era of social reform, the recognition

of health problems related to industrial development and urbanization created a resurgence of interest in governmental responsibility for meeting health needs. The focus was health insurance coverage. Collapse of these efforts is attributed to vehement opposition—due to the fact that the proponents of health insurance had neglected to consider and deal with the economic and idealogical interests of other groups that would be involved in this social innovation.

Federal government involvement with the broad spectrum of health issues did not emerge as a serious focus for action in the United States until the 1930s. Incremental efforts to develop a more coherent national health policy and protections for the citizenry were stimulated by both the private and public sectors.

Prior to the 1930s, the concept of national health policy development based on planning and implemented through a related series of federal, state, and local organizations was largely fostered in the private sector. Local government, in major metropolitan areas (particularly New York City), had also assumed responsibility for a wide range of health programs. During the 1930s the serious economic dislocations, caused by the depression, suggested a need for greater governmental assistance at all levels.

Passage of the Social Security Act of 1935 was surrounded by efforts to address related health issues. They crystallized in the report of the Interdepartmental Committee to Coordinate Health and Welfare appointed by President Franklin D. Roosevelt in 1935. A report, entitled "A National Health Program,"[2] was presented to a National Health Conference convened by the President in 1938. It recommended greatly increased government participation in the field of public health including federal health insurance.

Over the next 30 years, repeated attempts to implement these proposals failed in the Congress. It was not until the passage of the Social Security Amendments of 1965 (Medicare and Medicaid) that the federal government began to assume a major responsibility for payment of health services.

This political commitment at the federal level (i.e., passage of the Medicare and Medicaid legislation) and the resulting rapid increase in federal expenditures for health, reestablished a related federal concern for health planning. Initial federal involvement in health planning began with passage of the Hill-Burton Act in 1946.[3] This Act was designed to increase the availability of hospitals through new construction in areas of need. Since hospital construction had been limited during the period of World War II its aim was to compensate for apparent shortages. The program was administered primarily through state construction agencies working in cooperation with hospitals. In the late 1950s and early 1960s, local areawide facilities planning councils were established in various parts of the country, and community (including consumer) representation on these councils was developed.

Community Based Planning

In the early 1960s under federal mental health legislation, a nationwide effort to institutionalize community based planning for the development of mental health programs was also begun. Passage of the Regional Medical Program legislation in 1965[4] created state and local organizations that were expected to work toward the regionalization of health services for victims of heart disease, cancer, and stroke. Community involvement and support came predominantly from the fields of medicine and hospital administration although eventually consumer participation was also sought.

In 1966 the Partnership for Health Act[5] provided the basis for establishment of state and areawide comprehensive health planning agencies. These agencies were to concern themselves with long-range planning for mental, physical, and environmental health purposes and to function with consumer dominated boards and advisory councils. Questions related to the cost of health care were expected to be addressed.

P.L. 93–641, the National Health Planning and Resources Development Act of 1974,[6] combined elements of the Hill-Burton, Regional Medical Program and Comprehensive Health Planning legislation. Programs funded under old legislation were terminated. A new system of state and local health planning agencies was created. These agencies were required to provide for broadly representative governing bodies with consumers in the majority and with appropriate representation from major providers of health services. While the focus of the planning effort was expected to be broad, increased emphasis was placed upon cost containment and health services delivery.

Planning Issues

As one can see, federally sponsored health planning efforts have become increasingly complex and cost conscious. Consumer and provider participants have been expected to grapple with related issues. Consumers are expected to introduce a broader perspective of community health needs and resources but they are generally less well versed than providers on the issues. This has presented a series of increasingly difficult and sometimes frustrating tasks. These problems are often compounded by:

A lack of clarification of the consumer's role in the work of the agency

An absence of adequate consumer orientation and training

The limitations of health planning agency staff support for consumer activities

The timing and location of agency activities which are unsuited to the full involvement of consumer members

Some health planning agencies are beginning to address these issues. Centers for Health Planning are expected to encourage and support health planning agency efforts. But in the foreseeable future it appears that consumer participants engaged in the work of health planning agencies will be required to take concerted and aggressive action to insure that their needs and the needs of the broader community are properly considered and met.

Consumer Contributions to Planning

Many consumers have already made major contributions to health planning in this community through involvement on boards and committees of a wide range of community organizations including the HSA. To those of us in the federal government this evidence of commitment and effort are welcome and gratifying.

With the promise of some form of national health insurance, the next several years will be particularly important. Knowledgeable and active consumers should play a major role in shaping this future.

High levels of consumer interest and the insightfulness of the questions being asked by consumers suggest to me that the consumers are ready, willing, and able to meet the challenge.

References

1. Rosen, G. *A history of public health.* New York: MD Publications, 1958
2. Marmor, T. R. *The politics of medicare.* Chicago, Il.: Aldine Publications, 1970 p. 8.

3. U.S.Congress, Hospital Survey and Construction Act. P.L. 79–725, August, 1946. (Known as the Hill-Burton Act).
4. U.S. Congress, Heart, Cancer and Stroke Amendments. P.L. 89–239, October, 1965. (Known as the Regional Medical Programs).
5. U.S. Congress, Comprehensive Health Planning and Public Health Services Act of 1966. P.L. 89–749, November, 1966.
6. U.S. Congress, National Health Planning and Resources Development Act of 1974, P.L. 93–641, January, 1975.

Chapter 9

WORKSHOP SUMMARIES

Workshop 1: The Health Systems Agency of New York City Reviews a Cat Scanner Proposal: A Simulation

Panelists: Neil Heyman
Assistant Director, Queens HSA
Queens, N.Y.

Lois Nadler
Health Planner, Project Review, New York HSA

Major Karl Nelson
Associate Director, Booth Memorial Medical Center
New York, N.Y.

Oscar Rosenfeld, C.S.W.
Assistant Dean for Administration
New York University School of Social Work
New York, N.Y.

Catherine Wynkoop
Assistant Director, New York HSA
New York, N.Y.

This workshop simulated an HSA project review of Booth Memorial's 1976 application for a CT (computed tomography) scanner. The Booth Memorial-HSA experience was chosen for presentation because it was felt to be a model of project reviews, particularly for scanners. The presentation provoked the kinds of questions that should be asked by consumers at project reviews and considered by hospital staff before submission of applications.

Mr. Rosenfeld, who chaired the Comprehensive Health Planning (CHP) task force which wrote the scanner guidelines, described their criteria. The actual staff summary of the Booth application was discussed by Ms. Nadler.

This reenactment began with Major Nelson's defense of Booth's application before the HSA subcommittee. Major Nelson then left the workshop and the actual minutes of the HSA's executive session were read. Workshop participants questioned the mock subcommittee on both the Booth application and the certificate of need process. How would the public learn of application hearings? How can consumer participation in prospective planning for such costly technology be achieved? And how can the medically indigent be assured of access to sophisticated diagnostic equipment like the CT?

Questions directed to the Booth application revealed concern with opportunities for regional planning. How frequently does Booth submit utilization figures to HSA scrutiny? Is the scanner safe from planning regulations once it is in place?

Major Nelson acknowledged that there has been no reevaluation of the scanner. While the HSA could not withdraw the approval of need, it could block future applications.

Participants asked the panel why Sweden and England together had as many scanners as New York City. Panel members replied that New York City is a world center for medical activity. The panel believed that the CT would eventually become a routine diagnostic tool. A major concern of the workshop audience was whether the CT and technology similar to it was medically and economically efficacious or merely impressive to doctors, administrators, and hospital trustees.

Workshop 2: Health Planning, Medicaid and Who's at Risk for What: The New York City Health Systems Agency Considers an Out-of-Hospital Childbearing Center

A Simulation of an Actual Project Review

Moderator: Sarah Frierson
Member, Board of Directors, New York City HSA
New York, N.Y.

Panelists: Doris Haire
President, American Foundation for Maternal and Child Health, Inc.
New York, N.Y.

Marsha Hurst, Ph.D.
Board of Directors, Maternity Center Association
New York, N.Y.

Michelle Kahmi
Board of Directors, Maternity Center Association
New York, N.Y.

Ruth Watson Lubic, C.N.M.
General Director, Maternity Center Association
New York, N.Y.

Shirley Mayer, M.D.
First Deputy Commissioner, New York City Health Department

John Steen
Acting Assistant Director, Staten Island HSA

A simulation of the Maternity Center Association's (MCAs) 1977 project review led this workshop into a lively discussion about the need for primary care institutions and the HSA role in fostering the development of innovative services.

Mrs. Lubic read the MCA staff summary presented to the HSA which requested an extension of the Center's designation as an independent diagnostic and treatment center for maternity care. Mr. Steen, Dr. Mayer (representing the New York City Department of Health) and Ms. Frierson (representing the HSA) played out their respective roles as indicated in the minutes of the project review subcommitee. The reenactment revealed as much about the politics of alternative versus traditional health care interests as the actual mechanics of the review process.

At issue were the extent to which the Center's approach could be regarded as "experimental" and its failure, in the Health Department's eyes, to guarantee sufficient hospital back-up services. Mrs. Haire, arguing on behalf of MCA, refuted the notion that the MCA was any more "risky" than traditional hospitals. She cited evidence that hospitals' routine interventions and use of technology in the birth process often do more harm than good. Difficulty in providing back-up was presented by MCA as being related to lack of support for the Center by the New York City Health Department.

Questions on birthing practices, composition of staff, payment methods, and data collection at the Center were raised by the audience. Mrs. Lubic responded, speaking to the active role of the client in her own care, and the tie-ins with other facilities and practitioners. She emphasized that the MCAs approach was not "a-technological."

The HSAs role in encouraging alternatives in health care was discussed. HSA panel members pointed to the problems they faced in reviewing alternative programs: the absence of professional unanimity on critical questions; the defensiveness of both professionals and institutions when faced with consumer defection; and the needs of consumers for low-cost, primary care.

One audience member noted an inconsistency between the HSA's support of the MCA application and its official endorsement of the federal obstetrical guidelines which regard childbirth as a medical event, appropriate to tertiary care institutions. There was no response to this observation.

Workshop 3: Breast Cancer: Prevention, Detection, and Treatment

Moderator: Henry Patrick Leis, Jr., M.D.
Clinical Professor of Surgery and Chief, Breast Service
New York Medical College
New York, N.Y.

Panelists: John Boland, M.D.
Department of Radiotherapy
Mount Sinai School of Medicine
New York, N.Y.

Andrea Eagan
Member and writer for HealthRight, a woman's health education and consumer advocacy organization
New York, N.Y.

Guy Robbins, M.D.
Department of Surgery and Director of Cancer Control
Memorial Sloan-Kettering Cancer Institute
New York, N.Y.

Philip Strax, M.D.
Medical Director, Guttman Institute
Associate Clinical Professor, Department of Community and Preventive Medicine
New York Medical College
New York, N.Y.

Dr. Leis opened the workshop with a lecture and slide show on the patterns of occurrence of breast cancer in the United States. Statistically, the white, more affluent, nulliparous, older (55 plus) female groups have the highest incidence. However, breast cancer in blacks and women under 55 is increasing. He attributed the overall increase in cases partly to greater female longevity. Early diagnosis and other factors have improved posttreatment survival rates.

Dr. Strax stressed his concern with detection rather than therapy. The landmark Health Insurance Plan of Greater New York (HIP) study of 20 years ago proved the positive results of early detection. Mammography is indicated for women under 50 when symptomatic; others should have the test yearly. Dr. Strax claimed that the recent "commotion" over radiation risks was based on highly speculative evidence. Strax believes the benefits of mammography greatly outweigh the risks, especially since radiation doses are now extremely small. Mammography, he said, could save the lives of 12,000, versus the six cases of radiation-induced cancer that might emerge in 10 to 15 years. Most cancers in the Guttman Institute's Screening Program were discovered in asymptomatic women under 50. Dr. Strax believes this finding makes the best case for routine mammography.

Dr. Robbins spoke on the success of control and cure of breast cancers of different stages. He conceded that the issue of surgery remains confusing and outlined the uncertainty of cancer growth rates and the variables of lesion size and location.

Dr. Leis deplored the idea "sold" to women that radical mastectomy is unnecessary, calling it a concern for cosmetics.

Briefly the history of surgery and radiation in breast cancer treatment was traced. Dr. Boland demonstrated that the choice and result of either therapy was closely correlated with tumor size and involvement of the surrounding lymph nodes.

Ms. Eagan credited the women's movement with influencing present surgical patterns and behavior of providers in presenting options in treatment. She challenged Dr. Strax's position on the safety and effectiveness of routine mammography. It does not necessarily distinguish tumors that present dangers and women cannot be sure that all diagnostic centers have safe levels of radiation, Dr. Leis commented that it is very rare to get more than one rad exposure anywhere today. He also briefly discussed the value of chemotherapy.

WORKSHOP 4: HOW MUCH TECHNOLOGY IS NEEDED FOR AN EFFECTIVE EMERGENCY MEDICAL SERVICES SYSTEM—IS IT WORTH IT?

Moderator: Norma J. Goodwin, M.D.
President, Amron Management Consultants, Inc.
New York, N.Y.

Panelists: Kathleen Hunt
Research and Evaluation Specialist of the NYC Emergency Medical Services System

Emil Pascarelli, M.D.
Chief of Ambulatory Care

Beekman Downtown Hospital
New York, N.Y.

Judith B. Wessler
Consumer Health Advocate, MFY Legal Services
New York, N.Y.

Moderator Norma Goodwin posed the question: Is an Emergency Medical Service—with its data systems, new ambulances and trained personnel—cost-effective?

Dr. Pascarelli traced the history of emergency medical services from mere transportation to a hospital, through the training of ambulance drivers in first aid to the current philosophy of "bring the hospital to the patient" which sprang from advances in cardiology. It is difficult to evaluate the benefits of a sophisticated EMS because of the rapid development of emergency technology within the past decade, the rising cost of that equipment, and the use of trained paraprofessionals.

The Federal EMS Act of 1973 inspired a boom in emergency services. Now, money is running out and the EMS must be justified. Costs could be cut by marketing the system, but ultimately consumers will bear the costs. Self-care education for consumers could reduce unnecessary utilization.

Dr. Pascarelli enumerated the costs involved in a typical, new ambulance: hardware plus the cost of ambulance and base station personnel comes close to a quarter of a million dollars.

Does an EMS save lives? One statistical study shows positive immediate effects. However, survival rates three months following emergency treatment are the real indicators of cost-effectiveness.

Are EMS costs high because of profits anticipated by equipment manufacturere? Dr. Pascarelli replied that hardware cost is outweighed by the cost of health professionals. He suggested that profit motives by manufacturers would be scrutinized under a national health service.

Can consumers be educated to determine a real emergency? Yes, but a study of that aspect of EMS efficacy is considered a low priority.

Ms. Hunt shared knowledge gained as an evaluator of New York City's EMS. Absence of hard data as well as the variables of mortality and morbidity make it very difficult to establish evaluation criteria. Existing studies are equivocal. Paramedics may inhibit or enhance outcome. An EMS may or may not improve survival rates. Finally, there should be other indicators of cost-effectiveness besides mortality.

Ms. Wessler, one of the few consumers involved in the Manhattan Plan to coordinate ambulance and emergency rooms in Lower Manhattan, suggested a more rational approach to ambulance deployment and an end to competitiveness between ambulance services. A small percentage of the population is being targeted as potential EMS users. The service should be extended to burn cases, to cases of poisoning, to infants in distress. Ms. Wessler concluded that while sophisticated equipment was helpful, a patient's living conditions may well undo the positive effects of EMS treatment.

The workshop ended with a brief discussion of the "worried well." If providers and consumers each define pain and illness in different ways, who will determine the true emergency?

Part III

THE ECONOMICS OF MEDICAL TECHNOLOGY

As most consumers would exclaim, "Finally, we get around to the root of all evil—money!" This third conference of the series concentrated upon the economic aspects of medical technology in the health care delivery system. In addition to the hard cash factors, this conference reviewed the social costs, public accountability investments, regulatory enforcement costs, the cost of lost opportunities, and the costs of under- and overdiffusion of technology. In terms of rising health care costs, the last speaker in the morning session posed the question, "Is Medical Technology the Villain?"

Economic aspects of the use of medical technology in health care are most difficult to isolate above and beyond the dollar cost of the equipment and the personnel. Who determines the dollar value of a life saved through the use of technology? What criteria are used to set a monetary amount on the alleviation of pain and discomfort? How can a disability be equated with a dollar figure? What is a small toe worth? These are only a small sampling of questions that could be raised when trying to make a judgment about the economic costs and benefits of medical technology. Of course, these same questions could be asked on a larger scale from the community. Communities must determine relative values in order to set priorities. Which are more important, kidney dialysis centers or heart transplants?

Once the transition is made from thinking about the individual to the overall community, different values come into play in the decision-making process. While it would certainly be ideal to be able to fund all the technologic activities, it is apparent that the dollars are going to have to be divided up among many projects. These economic constraints demand that we make choices. Such choices will be based on personal and societal values, moral and otherwise. In addition, there will be estimates of the effectiveness and the safety of the medical technologies and perhaps a cost-benefit ratio. Weighing all these factors relative to today's major health problems has led some consumers to advocate the use of primary care alternatives to render direct care to people rather than the investment in high technology equipment for the benefit of a limited number of people. In effect, a decision of this nature could be condemming certain patients to death or disability because the technology would not be available when needed. Of course, a response would be forthcoming indicating that the technology was not really that good anyway and the patients benefited would have done so without the technology. This is not an easy predicament to squeeze out of by saying that you are both right. People's lives are at stake.

With the current stress on the containment of health care costs, another economic aspect relates to the legislative mandates calling for rate setting and regulatory controls on certain reimbursement programs. Federal government administrators have proposed that "caps" be placed on the amount of money that hospitals can charge for services. One federal regulation requires a maximum allowable cost for prescription drugs dispensed in federal health care programs. Medicaid, Medicare, and maternal and child health programs consume a tremendous bite out of the federal health care dollar. Essentially, the question is rather simple, "Should he who pays the piper call the tune?" This same philosophy could translate down into the state and local levels as consumers sit on health planning agencies and other governing bodies and are pressed to make decisions. Obligations of the consumer representative on an HSA may conflict with the advocacy role of supporting health care as a right for all.

An objective of this third conference was to broaden the dimensions of the consumers beyond the visible apparent dollar signs. Many direct and indirect economic aspects of the impact of medical technology on health care activities will have to be considered during the decision-making process.

Charlotte Muller opened the third conference with a talk on the social costs of medical technology. This implied that many people do not consider the social costs. Her opening question reflected that point by asking, "Do we know the price we pay?"

Social costs may be difficult to determine and are related to the fact that medical technology involves different actors with different interests. Inventors and developers are keenly interested in technical performance. Patients and physicians look for clinical results without harm. Those paying for the services want to be sure that the technology is recognized and approved by the appropriate professional bodies. Regulators and standards setters have to evaluate the good and the bad and come to a happy compromise. It should be apparent that varying interests will make for approaches to the use of the technology in health care activities at varying speeds and influences.

Closely allied to the fragmented interest groups is the nonsystematic measurement of costs and benefits. In today's health reimbursement picture this is complicated by the fact that benefits may be to parties A and B while the costs are assumed by parties C and D. Possible inhibitions to a true measure of costs include the loss of patients over time for follow-up, the lack of controlled trials when benefits appear obvious, the lack of including the services of family members rendering care at home or elsewhere and the contributions of other community members who may be involved in the health care picture. Often, there is no record that will indicate these costs or, even further, place a dollar value on the specific items.

Some research has been conducted on the relationship between medical technology and the income of physicians. Muller reported on the analysis of the financial incentive to physicians to order diagnostic tests for a patient. An internist in solo practice was the model for three different situations. In model A, the doctor ordered no tests; in model B a percentage of patients received five diagnostic tests; in model C higher percentages were assumed to get tested. As a result of adding the tests, net physician income rose from $32,000 for A to $55,000 for B and to $60,000 for C. A fourth example, model

D, assumed a group practice physician. A 12-channel blood chemistry was added to the five tests ordered in models B and C. This raised the net income for the doctor to $90,000 with the same percentages as in Model C. Thus, the incentive to order tests for patients was intensified under group practice. Rewards per minute of time for the test is high according to the payment schedules of third-party insurers for certain tests. Therefore, the covered patient does not object. Physicians can make up for smaller payment schedules for office visits with the added tests. Issues raised here relate to the equitable distribution of existing technology and the priorities for new technology so those not covered by insurance receive quality health care.

Muller discussed the case of the CT scanner in an effort to detail the side effects and ensuing cost factors. She noted that Medicare had already set dollar limits on the payments for scans. In addition, it is claimed that alternatives to CT scans may be safer and more effective in specific situations. Attention was called to the social costs of releasing the patient from the psychic strain of diagnostic surgery or other techniques that are involved in using the CT scanner.

In addition to explaining under- and over diffusion of medical technology, Muller talked about cost accounting: economic, social, and indirect. When screening, cost must be figured not only for each test performed but for each case discovered. Once discovered, the cost must be calculated for the follow-up required to modify the disease state. During the course of treatment, supportive social relationships may be disrupted by the heavy emphasis on specialization. Professionals working in certain areas, such as radiation therapy, may suffer emotional stress and be unable to work for periods of time. This is a cost that shows up in family care agencies and in welfare or unemployment figures. Indirect costs can be evaluated only in a rather limited fashion. Measurement on the quality of life leaves much to be desired. Situations in which these difficult cost measurements occur include multiple births resulting from fertility drugs, intensive care for premature infants, organ transplants, surgical insertion of synthetic materials inside the body, and intensive cardiac care. All these services involve high-level medical technology for which the cost accounting problems are obvious and the evaluation of benefits and risks highly subjective.

In closing, Muller contended that medical technology decisions tend to be provider oriented with an emphasis on the clinical-technical effects. Psychosocial effects are given low priority and are often not measured at all. Technology decisions also tend to be affluence oriented shortchanging the impoverished. Furthermore, Muller called for continuous updating of the evaulation of technology's costs and benefits in order to keep pace with improved methods of measurement and with the changing environment.

Ted Bogue discussed the public's involvement in the development of new technologies from the viewpoint of consumer advocates. Bogue identified four points relative to the public accountability issue as vital for consumers to consider:

Symptoms of accelerating emphasis on medical technology in health care delivery

Causes of this trend

Medical technology development as a resource allocation problem

Possible solutions to uncontrolled proliferation of medical technology

Symptoms include the increased costs, the questions about diffusion before the efficacy is known, the need to drum up patients to use the proliferating machines and the tendency of physicians to use the technology inappropriately. In addition, the risk factor is always present and the variance in usage is not correlated to health status changes.

Causes of this trend reflect the decisive fact that there is relatively unrestricted control by doctors over decisions to purchase new technology. Physicians, hospitals, and trustees appear to favor more intensive use of technology. Coupled with the willingness of third-party payers to reimburse for the use, new technology moves rapidly into everyday practice. Consumers exercise little influence over purchase decisions.

Resource allocation emphasizes the finite economic resources available and the values that society places on expending funds for medical technology. Considerations of trade-offs and cost-benefit analyses are common tools for decisions.

Possible solutions could involve changing the economic incentives for physicians and hospitals and increasing the public and governmental involvement in controlling the proliferation of medical technology.

Alan Brownstein continues with a discussion of the public interest relative to medical technology. While the rapid growth of new medical technology is noted, attention is also called to the lack of accountability and the missing elements of planning and coordination. Because of these deficits, Brownstein states that too much happened too soon, distribution problems occurred, and the economic impact was severe. Aside from the inflationary costs, there were benefits that were lost since the funds for technology could not then be used to deliver primary health care services.

In proposing a public interest approach to medical technology, Brownstein emphasizes the assessment process wherein the new technology is critically evaluated before its routine use. Relying on reports from the Office of Technology Assessment and recent federal legislation, a number of recommendations are made at the federal, state, and local level. One suggestion calls for a National Center for Health Care Technology.

In closing, Brownstein poses a compelling question, "The choice is simple and complex—will new technology be shaped to meet the public interest, or will public interest be shaped to accommodate new technology?"

Spiralling costs of medical care were traced historically by Herbert Hyman in Chapter 12 and he asked, "Is medical technology the villain?" Hyman cited three major contributing factors: the Hill-Burton Act of 1946 that stimulated hospital construction; the creation of the National Institutes of Health with their stimulation of medical research; the international space race that led to the application of space age technology to medical care. Add to these factors the American consumer's faith in the capacity of technology to cure illness and the result is a powerful combination to increase spending. At the same time, professional education integrated the new technology into existing teaching programs. This occurred for physicians and others and for a new breed: the medical technologist such as the radiologic assistant, cytotechnologists, and various physicians' assistants. Once included in the training program, the graduates tend to use the technology routinely. Of course, hospital trustees and insurance companies also played their roles; one, by competing with other hospitals to secure impressive technical equipment and the other by paying for the hospitals' technology through reimbursement.

Hyman listed four primary sources of funds to pay for the technology: public tax monies, private nonprofit insurance companies, private philanthropy, and individual out-of-pocket expenses. Almost 70 percent of the funds from these sources were used to cover increases in payroll and nonpayroll expenses. Inflation added another 20 percent, bringing the total for these three factors up to 90 percent of the increased expenditures. Increased use and population growth added much smaller amounts. Yet, despite the increased costs, the consumer's net cost in 1974 was about the same as in 1950. For that net expenditure, the consumer received better care in a newer facility with the latest medical technology. Why should the consumer complain?

If this is so, why has there been a reaction now to the high costs of health care? Three factors are cited by Hyman. He claimed that the oil embargo of 1974 knocked the economy off course with the higher energy costs, that unions engaged in more collective bargaining relative to health care benefits and the public lost their faith in the efficiency of all levels of government. Eventually, federal legislators moved to do something by passing a law that stressed cost containment and the development of a rational approach to the health care delivery system. Health planning and regulation were the key ingredients of the new law. Hyman commented on his evaluation of the efforts with attention to health planning and regulation through rate setting with specific examples in health service areas.

In concluding, Hyman proposed three strategies for consumers to ponder that may reduce costs while increasing health status. A medical strategy, a self-help strategy, and a community based strategy were proposed.

Factors in the medical strategy included the reorientation of medical and allied health education and the rationing of medical technology through the use of resource distribution guidelines aimed at regionalization.

By self-help, Hyman means individual action to achieve improved personal health. Hyman reported on a study which corelated seven specific health habits that increased life expectancy. If followed, these habits would reduce the risk of death from the three major killers in America today: heart disease, cancer and stroke.

Community strategies considered wide gauge programs such as water fluoridation to combat dental decay, immunization for children, health education for the public, development of mental health crisis centers, and the curtailment of hazards in the workplace.

Hyman's last sentence drives home his point, "Yet, more and more, the people are becoming the masters of their own well-being."

Workshops at this conference included two actual HSA project review simulations, one role-playing situation, and a seminar on hospital costs. All the workshops covered the economic impact of the medical technology under discussion including a burn unit, a cytogenetic laboratory, and a family practice unit.

In the session reenacting the HSA subcommittee review of a burn unit proposal, those who had participated in the actual review played the roles of the applicant and the subcommittee members. Particular attention was paid to the financial viability of the proposed unit which required a great deal of new construction. All acknowledged the need for the burn unit in the community. Although certain aspects were questionably viable, highly emotional testimony of burn victims swayed the subcommittee to approve the unit. This approval, however, was overruled by the full project review committee. Another investigation took place within the HSA Executive Committee and the burn unit was again turned down despite a good deal of special interest lobbying. However, a burn unit was still felt to be needed and the HSA solicited other applicants. Another proposal was approved and a burn unit was established in renovated facilities in a hospital.

In another workshop, panelists were assigned to play roles as members of the governing board of a voluntary nonprofit hospital. These board members were asked to consider the creation of a family practice unit and its implications for primary care. An expert family care physician testified before the board giving the rationale for establishing a family practice unit. Audience members were able to see and hear the political aspects of this situation that were an outgrowth of the battle for status among the various medical specialists and the hospitals' need to protect its own domain. Questions were asked of the panel and each participant explained his fictional stance in terms of the special interests represented. Attitudes of various panelists represented experiences in similar health care situations. At the end of the mock board meetings, a vote was taken and the board appointed a committee to study the proposal.

A 1977 proposal to establish a centralized prenatal cytogenetic diagnostic laboratory was reenacted in a workshop by the participants in the actual HSA process. In addition to the concerns over cost and efficiency, the dimensions of dehumanization and ethics were added. Furthermore, the audience pointed out problems that might arise due to social attitudes and prejudice toward infants with congenital defects. Examples of economic planning included group purchasing, the effective design of the laboratory, and the conversion of existing equipment.

Hospital costs with an emphasis on definitions of terms and a discussion of issues was the topic of another workshop. In this session a comparison was made with the economic trends of other industries to the health care industry. A Health Maintenance Organization (HMO) was cited an an example of a merger in industrial terms. While some audience members were distressed by the industrial comparison, it was pointed out that the profit-making, fee-for-service health care industry was attractive to investors seeking dividends on their monies. Distinctions were made between hospital costs and hospital charges. Indirect costs, such as the expenses incurred in the training functions of hospitals, were discussed. Interest was expressed in the profit motive in rising hospital costs. One panelist commented. "The health care mess could be partially solved by restructuring the system of delivery and removing the profit motive."

Chapter 10

THE SOCIAL COSTS OF MEDICAL TECHNOLOGY: DO WE KNOW THE PRICE WE PAY?

Charlotte Muller

In a biography about Denis Diderot,[1] the famous French philosopher and encyclopedist of the Enlightenement, his pamphlet of 1748 dealing with the long-standing division of territory in medicine is described. Diderot noted that surgeons could not express an opinion on the general medical aspects of a case. Physicians, who were both upper class and inheritors of a priestly status, were forbidden to shed blood or to use manual skills. Diderot denounced this split and argued for a single curriculum. He said, what disadvantage is there today in the same person's ordering and executing a bloodletting? Among other things, this incident illustrates that coordination of services is not very useful to the patient unless the technology is worth delivering.

Different Parties at Interest

As distinct from administrative technology in health systems, medical technology involves the application of scientific knowledge to patient care. Physical and chemical modalities and biological products may be used. We must view the range as including complex instrumentation in one-time interventions, linkage of the organism to artificial systems periodically or continuously (e.g., hemodialysis and pacemakers), and pharmacological interventions repetitively carried out by the consumer on prescription. Often the sophistication of the technology depends on the synthesis of different scientific disciplines.

Medical technology is allied closely with information devices and systems. Examples include the localization of lesions through computerized axial tomography and the production of mathematical readings to guide clinical decisions or to adjust the rate of application of any intervention without a human action. Presentation of patient status data to the clinician along with the relevant knowledge base for selecting an optimal action is an example of fine tuning of care based on an elaborate technology of data entry, classification, and highly selective retrieval.

Some medical technology requires so much capital that the resources of a large institution to acquire, house, maintain, and operate it are a necessity. Personnel with highly specialized competence are needed. In other cases, the technology is easily adapted to office practice.

A major problem of today's health care is that medical technology involves parties with different interests. Developers are keenly interested in technical performance, The practitioner-patient dyad is in the market for clinical results or effect without harm. Each member of the dyad has monetary concerns, the former wants revenue and the latter, who must meet all health needs within a budget, is evaluating the likelihood of benefit and the priority to be accorded to the particular intervention. A third party at interest, the payer, wants to be sure that the professions recognize the device, procedure, drug, etc. as legitimate. Regulators and standards setters want to know when and how to "smile at the good and frown at the bad" and to achieve an optimal rate of adoption throughout the system.

Costs and Benefits

Costs and benefits are not measured systematically and compared with cost, and they are not netted out in the same amounts. Benefits may be to parties A and B; the costs assumed by parties C and D. The first is a measurement or knowledge issue, the second is an impact or policy issue. Overcoming this fragmentation is essential in developing a technology policy that is socially best.

Failure to measure benefits and true costs of technology is partly due to time problems. Over time, patients are lost from view; other life events cloud causal association. Another problem is the classic ethical dilemma in the design of sufficiently controlled trials when benefit appears very obvious. Still another difficulty in assessing technology is that the undervaluation of the needs and contributions of certain segments of society according to deeply entrenched biases distorts measurement. An example is return of a patient to the home having undergone a massive intervention and now dependent on unpaid ministration of a wife who is prevented from taking part in market or nonmarket activities. Services of the family member do not get accounted for and the condition and outcome are measured for the patient exclusively. Some of these flaws do yield to more advanced evaluation approaches and others to evolution of social attitudes, such as concern with what happens to well women taking a contraceptive medication for decades of the fertile period.

Physician Income and Technology

A mixture of more and less established technologies in ambulatory care is considered in an interesting recent study by Schroeder and Showstack.[8] They analyzed the financial incentive to physicians to order diagnostic services for a patient. Eight tests were considered, including the electrocardiogram, the sigmoidoscopy, and the 12-channel blood chemistry analysis. While the direct financial incentive is not the only factor, being reinforced by doctors' training, patient expectations, and desire to avoid malpractice suits, the example as developed shows the power of the cash incentive.

An internist in solo practice is the model with the space, workload, expenses, and relative values for different services under the California Relative Value Studies detailed, following reasonable assumptions. In Model *A*, the doctor orders no tests. But in Model *B*, 40 percent of patients coming for an initial or comprehensive visit and 7 percent of those coming for a routine return visit get an electrocardiogram, and other percents are applied to four other tests: urine, complete blood count, sigmoidoscopy, and tuberculosis skin test. In Model *C*, higher percents are assumed to get tests. Fewer patients are seen in Models *B* and *C* compared to *A* in order to allow realistically for the time needed to do and read tests. As a result of adding the tests, net income is raised from under $32,000 with no tests in Model *A* to $55,000 in Model *B* and $60,000 in Model *C*.

As developed in Model *D*, the fourth case is a group practice where equipment and space are shared. A variety of tests are done for the same proportions of patients as in Model *C* but the 12-channel blood chemistry and two other tests are added. This raises the net income per doctor to $90,000. Thus, the incentive to test is intensified under group practice.

Basically, the incentive to test is that the reward per minute of time for the tests is very high in the payment schedule used by third-party insurers, while for tests such as x-ray the marginal cost of equipment use is low once the equipment is in place. Furthermore, the patient does not object because direct obligation to pay is limited. In addition, the authority of the physician interacts with the patient's fear of illness and the desire to recover. Under certain payment schemes, doctors who order a variety of tests are able to make up for the ceiling on the allowed charge for the visit itself. Regulatory mechanisms such as Certificate-of-Need (CON) programs and Professional Standard Review Organizations (PSROs) do not object to test proliferation in ambulatory care because they have, by and large, been confined to hospitalization norms. Physicians make their own guidelines because the efficacy of tests in changing the course of treatment has been evaluated insufficiently even for, or perhaps especially for, established technologies. Or else the physician has not read, or has chosen not to follow, the literature.

For those patients who are deterred by the residual charge —for example, the copayment under Medicare of 20 percent of the allowed charge—the technology, whether needed or not, has remained inaccessible. Hence, one of the issues raised by the exposition of incentives in the Schroeder and Showstack model is the equitable distribution of existing technology. Another issue is the equitable determination of priorities for areas of new technologies so that the health problems of the disadvantaged are addressed.

Hospitals and Technology

It has been calculated that a large share of the increase in hospital costs in recent decades is due to new technology.[3] Most innovation has been directed toward creating new health care products rather than increasing efficiency with which the old are produced. While this is commonplace in the history of technology in society, it became an explosive issue in health care because inflation, labor-intensive hospital production, popularity of hospitals, and other factors made the efficiency problem important. In addition, a general cap on hospital costs relative to national income became a major policy question. Incentives for technology advances within hospitals lie within complex interrelations among scientific developers, capitalists, physicians, hospital boards and administrators, and patients. A potential gain that is often realized are positive capabilities added in the diagnosis and treatment of disease. Open heart surgery, pacemakers, and new drugs have made survival, activity, and comfort possible for those previously condemned to other fates. Yet, costs and consequences must still be considered in allocating social resources.

CT Scanners

As an example, the CT scanner is worth some discussion. Used to produce high quality images of soft tissue structures, the technology of CT scanning was started in England and took root rapidly in the United States within the last five years. It was adopted in head scans before its diagnostic efficacy could really be studied and certainly before its implications for treatment and outcome could be traced. It was also introduced in body scans. In 1977, the Institute of Medicine (IOM)[4] considered that evidence as to the effect on other diagnostic steps and hospitalization could not be called adequate. Thus, CT scanning became a prototype for the adoption of technology for privately rational motives without protection of the public resource pool. Responsibility for this movement has been given to:

1. Interhospital competition for revenue, staff, and image
2. Reimbursement that removes risk from investment
3. Perverse effects of CON programs on early adoption to avoid risk or denial
4. Fee opportunities for physicians

In addition, our medical culture values tests, rewards their application, and punishes their omission. A charge on reimbursement systems results.

In order to conduct a full evaluation of efficacy, risks must be considered. The IOM committee noted risks of allergic reactions to injected contrast materials (used in about 60 percent of scans). While risks of ionizing radiation are less than for invasive x-ray procedures, continued study in comparison with other imaging methods was recommended.

Changes in design are rapid and tests of efficacy based on earlier, slower scanners became obsolete. Yet, the enthusiasm and interest of leading practitioners has continued. A reimbursement policy consistent with this state of affairs is authorization for payment in settings that are part of a clinical trial. While reimbursement systems have not yet required clinical trials to authorize payment for diagnostic tests, Medicare already requires entering certain diagnoses as a condition for payment for scans and limits the allowed charge to $150.

Whether a clinical trial rule will greatly check disbursements cannot be predicted. For serious head conditions and in the presence of invasive alternative strategies, a CT scan may have a highly inelastic demand. For body scanning, more negotiability is present, but the list of appropriate uses is growing. It is claimed by the IOM, however, that the CT scan is not superior to alternatives in all uses (ultrasonic imaging is safer in obstetrics and provides better information in cardiology). While the evaluation literature on the scanner continues to grow, there remains a divergence of aims between practitioners and hospitals interested in an additional use at low marginal cost to them, and the reimbursement and public health authorities interested in limiting location and use of scanners. Requiring certain professionals on staff, and limiting locations to institutions able to treat the diagnosed conditions, are among the suggested controls.

Capital costs of an evolving technology usually drop after the early stages as efficient production approaches are worked out and competition operates. Also, the fee for professional services may drop as skills are learned outside a narrow range of subspecialists. Therefore, the fear of imposing a heavy cost on the system based on the price of the first round of scanners is not fully justified. It is not easy, however, to project costs of operation from existing locations. Furthermore, in 1977 the IOM believed that both the charges for doing the scan and the physician fees for reading it were high relative to inputs used. In overall assessment of net social costs of CT scanning, the release from the psychic strain of diagnostic surgery, pneumoencephalography, etc. should be included. At the same time, any new technique has potential for mischief if findings are transmitted that sound ominous to patients but are not of current clinical significance.

Underdiffusion and Overdiffusion

Living with technology involves several classes of problems. Underdiffusion was once a real worry to health care policy makers. This yielded to overdiffusion as health care led the inflationary trend of our economy as any waste posed a major block to resource use to improve equity of accesss. Specifically, technology may be deemed overused since the health benefits of an innovation may not be demonstrated with certainty, the side effects may wipe out gains in the recognition and treatment of the primary disease, and the technology while generically valid may be applied to the wrong patients. Overdiffusion, moreover, does not preclude underdiffusion. An innovation may not reach those who could benefit by it because of controls imposed to prevent excessive adoption. CON controls could prevent installation of a CT scanner in a facility serving trauma victims in a low-income area, because another institution already has the equipment.*

We have become aware of medical side effects of technology such as serious gastric ulcer following antiarthritic medication. An economic side effect not too well explored is the use of technology as competitive advantage to a network of practitioners who have access to it. For example, a referral for a colonoscopy or gastrocopy using new fiberoptic techniques may have to come from a doctor on the staff of a hospital where the endoscopy exists. There is also reason to believe that the fee

*In this instance, there was another hospital scanner in the same metropolis and still others were in private offices. There were serious logistic problems in doing the scans and completing diagnoses efficiently.

structure for the services urgently demanded represents monopoly elements, with the limit being the cost of alternative modalities, rather than the cost of producing the services. In old railroad trust terms, this is charging what the market will bear.

Cost Accounting: Economic, Social, and Indirect

In accounting for the cost of technology to society, the impact on detection and treatment of disease must be assessed. For disease detection technology, one must consider the cost not just for each test performed, but per case found and confirmed. This means a reckoning based on natural prevalence in a population; the cost of acquiring, installing, and running a test capacity; the percent of capacity that will be used normally (which captures duplication's effect); and the cost of steps undertaken to deal with false positives. Costs of false negatives missed (the price of other detection steps that must be used or the cost of the progression of the undetected disease) must not be omitted. Highly sophisticated research models are being applied to this class of problems. Results are not easy to interpret.

Cost accounting must also assess the possibility of modifying the course of disease after it is found, including anatomic and physiological modification and functional restoration. Successful repair of nerve endings without being able to raise motor capacity high enough to remove gross dependency will not change either the psychosocial or the financial impact of disease. Life expectancy may be unaffected by exquisite techniques for disease identification. A partial technology may eventually be supplemented by the other pieces that would make a decisive difference. To keep certain activities going against this day may be a legitimate investment. More immediately, the fact that a new diagnostic technology allows avoidance of invasive, expensive, and otherwise undesirable diagnostic modalities to which patients are subjected may make it possible to show medical and economic gain even if ultimate outcome is unaffected.

Technology sets barriers in the way of supportive social relationships in the presence of disease and adds its own strains to the existing ones. One of these is that specialization is intensified and the patient and family do not always know where information, counseling, and responsibility are to be found. The life of the practitioner is altered too. A recent report from the Los Angeles press[5] cites a drop in productivity among certain radiation therapists who are emotionally unable to put in a full year's work even though they have various individual strategies of disinvolvement. Another example is a person undergoing mammography who can return for years without ever meeting the mammographer-physician face-to-face. How does she get help in interpreting disquieting reports about the dangers in the technique? Is this implicated in the observed drop in utilization and the loss of protection for considerable numbers of women?

Our modes of evaluating indirect costs are rather limited. Economic losses due to years of morbidity or premature death can be measured if certain assumptions are followed as to labor force participation and appropriate wage rates. In addition, the reasonableness of projecting present statistics rather far into the future has to be accepted. This information can be used to estimate losses that are averted by new treatments and losses caused by side effects. It is of little use for the retired and those producing nonmarket services. Another approach studies costs of alternative technologies per year of life gained, but the necessity of adjusting for quality of life to some extent brings in through the back door the allowance for economic productivity. Measurement of the impact on the quality of life has a long way to go. There is not yet an adequate conceptualization of the exchanges of services occurring in human network of kin and friends and how they are distorted by technologies. Only a small portion of this is captured by work loss measurements.[6] We have no reimbursement methods for supportive and counseling services to families of patients and consequently cannot even measure what services appropriate to the problems generated by the application of technology would have cost. Situations to which these remarks apply include: multiple births after using fertility drugs, surviving premature infants, organ transplant, drugs with behavioral side effects, detection of asymptomatic disease, surgical insertion of synthetic materials inside the body, dialysis, and intensive cardiac care.

High Technology Alternatives

An absence of collective societal responsibility for health maintenance as a full-bodied alternative to encapsulated pursuit of high technology activities in health care is a central problem in American health care. This absence is felt in the inadequacies of the structural context in which innovation is diffused. Decisions are typically provider-oriented. Psychosocial effects are given lower rating than clinical-technical effects, and often are not registered within the health care system. Difussion of technology is also affluence-oriented. Providers in poverty areas may not capture the new technology before diffusion is controlled. Finally, evaluation over time is not built into our health care system. Moreover, evaluation of technology's benefits and costs needs updating because of continuous development of the discipline of evaluation studies and the changing environment in which the technology is applied. For example, a person over 65 who is employed has a different biological equilibrium and profile from one who is not. Also, evaluation of preventive strategies should be as disciplined as assessment of high technology approaches to health problems.

Thermography illustrates the need for better evaluation of medical technology as a guide to diffusion and appropriate use. A report in the *New England Journal of Medicine*[7] refers favorably to thermography as a helpful method of pinpointing early breast cancers and states that it "assumes considerable priority in breast cancer detection if it is available." This same report also speaks well of xeroradiography as a method that "has much to offer in the early detection of breast cancer." That article was dated July 9, 1970. Since it was written, medical opinions have changed and evaluative techniques have also changed. Thermography has lost its following. More generally, giving of advice to clinicians as to the choice of techniques is now recognized to require a more complicated decision strategy based on mathematical analysis.

Solutions to problems related to medical technology should be based on recognition of technology and science as powerful social resources, if adequate social controls are applied.

References

1. Wilson, A. M. *Diderot.* New York: Oxford University Press, 1972, pp. 92–93.
2. Schroeder, S. A., & Showstack, J. G. Financial incentives to perform medical precedures and laboratory tests: Illustrative models of office practice. *Medical Care,* 1978, *16* 289–298.
3. Gaus, C. R., & Cooper, B. S. Technology and medicare: Alternatives for change, in R. H. Egdahl & P. M. Gertman (Eds.). *Technology and the quality of health care.* Germantown, Md.: Aspen Systems Corp., 1978. Estimates for 1967–1976 attribute 47 percent of the increase in community hospital expense per diem to new technology.
4. Institute of Medicine. *A policy statement, computed tomographic scanning.* Washington, D.C.: National Academy of Sciences, 1977.
5. Freed, K. How Doctors Deal with Cancer. *The Bergen Record,* October 1, 1978 from the *Los Angeles Times.*
6. An authoritative compilation of national statistics on diabetes does not present any estimates on the impact of diabetes on family members either in terms of frequency or in terms of dollar values nor does it even refer to such effects as something to be considered in assessing socioeconomic costs. DHEW Pub. No. (NIH) 78–1468, Diabetes Data Compiled 1977. Washington, D.C.: U.S. Government Printing Office, 1978.
7. Gershon-Cohen, J., Hermel, M. B., & Murdock, M. G. Priorities in breast cancer detection. *New England Journal of Medicine,* 1970, *283*, 82–85.

Chapter 11

DEVELOPING NEW MEDICAL TECHNOLOGIES

How and Why the Public Should Be Involved

Ted Bogue

An increasing share of the health care dollar, and indeed of the entire economy, is being devoted to medical technology. Therefore it is essential that resources be allocated to such technology in a way which is accountable to the general public.

Four features of this issue must be considered by consumers who wish to enhance the benefits and control the costs of medical technology to society:

1. The symptoms of accelerating emphasis on medical technology in health care delivery
2. The causes of this trend
3. The need to look at medical technology development as a resource allocation problem
4. Possible solutions to the apparent uncontrolled proliferation of medical technology

SYMPTOMS

What observations can one make about the world of medical technology? First, the cost is high and increasing in both absolute and relative terms. It is possible that we will soon be spending about one billion dollars annually on both computerized tomography scanning[1] and on coronary bypass operations.[2] From 1967 to 1976, hospital costs per patient day increased from $49 to $147. Researchers have estimated that $46 or 47.3 percent of this increase was due to increased "intensity" of services beyond general inflation, essentially new medical technology and associated costs.[3]

Second, the quality or efficacy of new medical technology is usually unknown before it is diffused into the health care delivery system. When efficacy is evaulated, particularly with regard to diagnostic tests such as CT scanning, health outcomes are not examined. Studies look at the quality of CT scanner images, not at whether CT leads to changes in therapy or improved health. Consequently, we often do not know whether we are better off with the technology (or with as much as we have) than without it.

Third, machines often proliferate so quickly that not enough patients can be found to make use of all the available capacity. This has been true of open heart surgery units and other equipment such as autoanalyzers, diagnostic x-ray machines, and patient monitors.[4]

Fourth, at the same time, doctors who make use of the technology tend to use it inappropriately, in part to retrospectively justify the need for it. Roemer's law says that hospital beds which are built tend to be used. Roemer's law also holds for medical technology: machines that are purchased tend to be used. This leads to a syndrome which might be called "if it's good for anyone, it must be good for everyone." For example, substituting CT scans for invasive procedures such as cerebral arteriograms and pneumoencephalograms, which are often painful and risky, is desirable. But we now have the capacity to do nearly three million scans a year.[5] Procedures being replaced never accounted for more than 400,000 tests a year.[6] Only 13 percent of the CT capacity would be necessary for total replacement of these two invasive procedures.

Fifth, there is no such thing as risk-free technology. We always run the risk of the therapy being more dangerous than the disease which is being treated. One of the most disturbing examples was the gastric freezing machine for duodenal ulcers. This machine was widely used for a few years in the early 1960s and then abandoned because it proved to be valueless and to have serious adverse side effects.[7]

Sixth, the use of medical technology and other therapies varies dramatically from one setting to another, without corresponding differences in health status. Tonsillectomy rates varied tenfold among hospital service areas within the state of Vermont.[8] Hospital utilization rates are much higher in the Northeast than they are on the West coast.[9] Medicaid surgery and hospitalization rates are more than twice as high among fee-for-service providers as among health maintenance organizations.[10]

CAUSES

There are many reasons for the diffusion of expensive medical technology of unproven value. The reasons are all related to one central fact, however, that of relatively unrestricted control by doctors over decisions to buy and use the equipment. This is manifested in several different ways.

First, consumers exercise little influence over the purchase and use of technologic serivces. Consumers are told very little about the actual costs, risks, and benefits of medical therapies. People tend to defer to doctors in deciding what health services to use. Individuals are encouraged to use new medical technology by the tendency of the mass media to glamorize the so-called miracles of modern medicine. Furthermore, consumers are discouraged from being cost-conscious by insurance coverage which is more complete for more expensive and technologic services. Even the insurance premiums are often paid by the employers. Resulting higher prices and taxes and lower wages are not linked in the consumer's mind with his or her use of health services.

Second, every incentive facing doctors, the real decision makers, favors more intensive use of technology. All the technologic equipment and specialized personnel in hospitals are used by doctors rent-free. Use of physician-owned technology (e.g., CT scanners) and performance of hospital based procedures (such as surgery) is often personally profitable for the physician. Medical education glorifies technological, hospital-oriented specialities. Doctors in such specialties also earn more. Professional prestige and rewards seem to be directly proportional to the intensity and specialization of the technology used by the physician. Thus, neurosurgeons are high in the medical pecking order and family practitioners are low. Finally, malpractice litigation encourages "defensive medicine," the use of all types of technology by physicians to avoid law suits.

Third, hospitals have similar protechnology incentives. Although hospitals are technically nonprofit, they need revenue to expand and modernize. Hospitals get revenue from patients (or their insurers) indirectly by attracting physicians to the hospital medical staff. By catering to their professional desires, hospitals attract and keep physicians in line with the incentives just discussed; professional desires tend to run toward high technology, specialized services. This technology is compounded by the propensity of hospital administrators and trustees to try to enhance the hospital's prestige by building more and more physically impressive facilities. All of this creates expansionist, "bigger is better" hospitals. And, as Professor Roemer pointed out, once hospitals have the facilities, they must use them in order to raise enough revenue through fee-for-service reimbursement to pay the purchase cost. A study of Boston hospitals lends empirical support to this view of hospital purchases of medical technology.[11]

Fourth, the third-party payers, Blue Cross and Blue Shield, the commercial health insurers, and the government through Medicare and Medicaid have historically been willing to pay for virtually whatever the doctors and hospitals want. Attempts to restrict this free flow of money by third parties and government through reimbursement and utilization controls and health planning have nearly always been taken over or neutralized by the health care industry. Major purchasers—unions and employers—have only recently begun to realize the need for controlling costs by controlling providers.

A net result of all these factors is a market of virtually unlimited financial potential for manufacturers of medical equipment. Providers have an insatiable appetite for more technology and the third parties (and ultimately the public) will pick up the bill without asking many questions.

Resource Allocation

One way to introduce some rationality into the medical technology spiral is to think in terms of resource allocation. Several propositions then become evident.

First, we do not have infinite economic resources. Every dollar we spend on new medical technology is a dollar we cannot spend on other kinds of goods and services, either inside or outside the health care sector.

Second, health care expenditures are limited only by the amount of money that the society is willing to spend on it. New medical technology and services can be created by the health care industry to absorb any number of additional dollars or any percentage of the gross national product.

Third, therefore we are forced to make trade-offs among competing objectives: between health care and other social programs such as housing, food, welfare, and education, and, within the health care sector, between high technology, institutional care, and primary, emergency, and preventive care or improved access to services in underserved areas.

Ideally, we should try to assess the costs, risks and benefits of all medical technology and therapies and spend development funds on those which seem most promising. Indeed, some *existing* high technology services with low benefits and high costs (such as excess surgery or CAT scanners) would be replaced by other health or social services which are more cost beneficial in terms of social welfare.

SOLUTIONS

There are two sets of strategies that might make the development of medical technology more publicly accountable: changing the economic incentives facing doctors and hospitals, and increasing public and governmental involvement in the development and proliferation of medical technology.

Economic Market Approaches

Generally the most consistently successful method of controlling utilization of medical technology and health services has been Health Maintenance Organizations (HMOs). Two keys to HMO cost control include the prepayment of a fixed annual amount for a comprehensive range of services and the use of salaried physicians who are rewarded for controlling utilization. Because the HMO has a fixed budget, it is forced to control use of the most expensive, high technology services in order to avoid losing money. As discussed above, HMOs hospitalize and operate on their patients much less frequently. Evidence also suggests that HMOs make more rational use of technology.[12]

In HMOs, the patient or his payer do not pay on a fee-for-service basis. As a result, HMOs have no economic incentive to provide a high volume of services. Payment systems can also be arranged so that patients are financially rewarded for choosing a more efficient delivery system. Anticompetitive restrictions from both organized medicine and government policy must be removed in order to allow natural HMO expansion.

Competitive pressures created by the HMO strategy have many advantages. They lead to putting doctors at financial risk for their own decisions to buy or use medical technologies and forcing them to do their own cost-benefit analysis. HMOs create a market for cost cutting rather than cost-increasing technology. This, in turn, has an effect on research and development priorities by medical equipment manufacturers and government.

Public and Governmental Regulation

Market incentives may go far toward more rational development and diffusion of medical technology, but alone they may be insufficient. Also, they cannot be created immediately. Direct public regulation may also be in order. Several alternative approaches have been suggested, and some are already in place.

Federal government agencies are now considering more formal ways to assess biomedical research priorities as well as the development and proliferation of medical technology, at least with regard to government-funded programs. Unfortunately, lay consumer involvement is generally weak. Consumers are more directly involved in Health Systems Agencies in determining the introduction and placement of medical equipment at the local level. Health planning could be strengthened by developing a capital expenditures budget that would limit the total amount of new equipment purchased. Some national health insurance proposals have an overall budget for all costs, labor as well as capital, again forcing decision makers to make trade-offs between technology and other services. Preauthorization for catastrophic health expenses has been proposed. Finally, third parties such as Blue Cross and Medicare could refuse to reimburse for unproven technology.

REFERENCES

1. Bogue, T. D., & Wolfe, S. M. *CAT scanners: is fancier technology worth a billion dollars of health consumer's money?* Washington, D.C.: Public Citizen Health Research Group, 1976.
2. Ross, R. S. Testimony given before the Senate Subcommittee on Health and Scientific Research of the Human Resources Committee. Hearings on Oversight of Biomedical and Behavioral Research in the United States, 1977, Part 3, p. 12.
3. Gaus, C. R., & Cooper, B. S. Technology and medicare: alternatives for change, in R. G. Egdhal & P. M. Gertman (eds.) *Technology and the quality of health care.* Germantown, Md.: Aspen Systems Corp., 1978.
4. ABT Associates. *Incentives and decisions underlying hospitals' adoption and utilization of major capital equipment.* Prepared for the National Center for Health Services Research and Development. September, 1975, pp. 100–109.
5. Bogue & Wolfe, see note 1.
6. Office of Technology Assessment. *Policy implications of the computed tomography (CT) scanner.* Washington, D.C.: U.S. Govt. Printing Office, 1978, p. 34.
7. Fineberg, H. V. *Gastric freezing: diffusion of a medical innovation.* Testimony given before the Senate Subcommittee on Health and Scientific Research of the Human Resources Committee. Hearings on Oversight of Biomedical and Behavioral Research in the United States, 1977, Part 3, pp. 46–63.
8. Wennberg, J. & Gittelsohn, A. Small area variations in health care delivery. *Science,* 1973, *182,* 1102–1108.
9. Griffith, H. R., & Chernow, R. A. Cost effective acute care facilities planning in Michigan. *Inquiry,* 1977, *14,* 229, 230.
10. Gaus, C. R., Cooper, B. S., & Hirschman, C. G. Contrasts in HMO and fee-for-service performance. *Social Security Bulletin,* 1976 *39* (5), 3, 9.
11. ABT Associates, see note 4, pp. 225–230.
12. Schroeder, S. A., & Showstack, J. A. *The dynamics of medical technology use: analysis and policy options.* Health Policy Program, School of Medicine, University of California, San Francisco, 1977, p. 40.

DEVELOPING NEW MEDICAL TECHNOLOGIES

Medical Technology and the Public Interest

Alan P. Brownstein

Medical technology includes the "drugs, devices, and medical and surgical procedures used in medical care, and the organizational and supportive systems within which such care is delivered."[1] Medical technology has been the major force shaping medical care since the 1950s. According to government officials, it is directly or indirectly responsible for 50 percent of the increase in costs of hospital care from $13.2 billion in 1965 to $40.9 billion in 1974. Almost 70 percent of medical technology research development is financed by government dollars. Despite the magnitude and importance of medical technology, there is serious question as to whether the process for the development and introduction of new technology into the mainstream of the health care delivery system best serves the public interest.

Lack of Accountability

Although research and development (R & D) is funded largely by the public sector, there is little public involvement in decisions concerning R & D priorities and the dissemination of medical technology. The major source of funding for biomedical research is from the National Institutes of Health (NIH) of the Department of Health, Education, and Welfare (HEW).

The NIH is comprised of 11 semiautonomous institutes organized around specific disease categories (e.g., cancer), organs (e.g. heart, lung), or age.

These institutes formed 52 peer review "study sections" comprised of outside scientists who specialize in these areas. NIH funding priorities and decisions are derived largely from the recommendations of these study sections which assess proposals for funding based on "scientific merit." Grant proposals for funding are also reviewed by the National Advisory Councils, which include some lay members, and are attached to each institute. But their recommendations generally follow those of the study sections.

Scientific merit alone is insufficient for the assessment of medical technology. Most NIH monies are awarded to private institutions (largely academic) to support R & D activities, initiated and proposed by individual scientists. With "scientific merit" as the major criterion for funding research, there is little room for a coordinated research strategy organized around goals and objectives that would best serve the public interest. Thus, only a portion of NIH funds are targeted towards achieving progress in specific areas. Under the rationale of "scientific merit," most NIH funds are distributed in a random haphazard fashion. Too often the public interest is served by accident, rather than by design.

Lack of Planning and Coordination

Medical technology brought about many important advances in combating human disease. Such was the case with the introduction of antibiotics in the 1940s and 1950s. Antibiotics proved to be safe, effective, and inexpensive. New vaccines have done much to reduce the incidence of measles and the dreaded disease, poliomyelitis. Diseases such as pneumonia and tuberculosis now require shorter hospital stays as a result of new medication.

However, there is another side to medical technology. All new technology does not provide miracles. Much of today's new technology is characterized as "half-way technology," which merely palliates the "manifestations of major diseases whose underlying mechanisms are not yet understood and for which no definitive prevention, control or cure has yet been devised."[2] Compared with the more definitive technologies, half-way technologies (e.g. organ transplants, renal dialysis) are the most expensive and provide the least benefit to the individual. New technology is too frequently introduced into the health care delivery system with insufficient evaluation as to its effectiveness, cost, appropriate use, safety, and other dimensions of impact. Planning is not done prospectively, before the dissemination of a new technology, but instead retrospectively, after much of the technology has been introduced inappropriately into the system; this is frequently too late. It is easier to prevent errors of dissemination before the fact, rather than trying to erase past errors that have become fixed in large capital investments and medical practice. The National Health Planning and Resources Development Act (P. L. 93-641) specifically prohibits Health Systems Agency (HSA) review of R & D activity. Section 1513 (e) reads that "HSA *shall not* review and approve or disapprove the proposed use within its health service area of funds appropriated for (research) grants or contracts . . . unless the grants or contracts are to be used to support the development of health resources intended for use in the health service area." Again, this is too late. From the experience in New York City, even research grants or contracts with health service or delivery implications are rarely, if ever, reviewed even though the HSA has authority to do so.

Coordination is also lacking. In addition to the NIH there

are no less than 8 other agencies within HEW and 11 federal agencies outside of HEW that are involved in health research that are all unconnected. Development of diagnostic ultrasound involved 19 separate agencies budgeted in their own orbits and is a good illustration of this fragmentation.

The private sector also funds research and development activity, mainly in applied research. While contributing less than one-third of the research dollar, the private sector has the role of introducing technology into the marketplace, directed by the profit motive, not health needs or priorities. For example, American Home Products, which manufactures Sani-Flush, also produces and markets fetal monitors. The lack of public accountability, planning, and coordination, created a number of undesirable effects in the introduction of new technology:

1. *Too Much Technology (Too Soon).* Premature, inadequately regulated introduction of medical technology into the health care delivery system resulted in duplication, misuse, and overuse. Mammography was widely accepted and used by the medical profession before important questions about its safety were addressed. Fetal monitors are commonplace in obstetric units throughout the United States. Yet, many of those who use this new technology neither understand when its use is appropriate, nor do they fully understand how to interpret fetal monitor readings. It is said that this misuse and overuse had led to a major increase in caesarean sections that were not necessary. Coronary bypass surgery is now performed 70,000 times per year. Yet, studies have shown that for most types of patients, this relatively new and expensive surgical procedure has not resulted in extended life span. Some estimates suggest that as little as 10 percent of all procedures now used in medical practice have been shown to be effective by controlled studies.

2. *Problems in Distribution of New Technology.* Whether or not the benefit of a new technology is clearly established, there are serious problems associated with the distribution of new technology. In Massachusetts, for example, computerized

axial tomography (CAT) scanners were housed in six teaching institutions in Boston in the early 1970s. The CAT scanner was widely accepted and desired by other hospitals in Massachusetts even though there was no clear-cut understanding of its effect on health status. Yet, at that time, it was determined that there were a sufficient number of CAT scanners in Massachusetts, and the Certificate-of-Need agency rejected an application for a CAT scanner from a hospital many miles from Boston. It is understandable that the major medical centers and medical schools would have initial access to new technologic equipment in the R & D stage, but this also precludes the potential for a rational regional distribution of new technology. Clearly, there has got to be a better way.

3. *Economic Impact.* Traditional economics cannot be applied to health care. Basic principles of supply and demand do not work because of the following reasons:

Most of the bills are paid by public and private insurers, not the person who benefits from the services, i.e., the patient.

The provider, i.e., physician triggers the demand for services.

Our social value system places a higher premium on health care than it does on many other social goods and services.

These economic imperfections are most dramatic in medical technology. Lewis Thomas[3] states that "in medicine, it is characteristic of technology that we do not count the cost, ever, even when the bills start coming in." Geiger[4] observed that "There is no 'effective demand among American consumers for a barium enema or a heart-valve repair, and there is no free market' for hospital rooms as there is for hotel rooms. You don't get them at all without a physician's order: but when a physician orders them, you almost always get them. The suppliers control, even create, the demand."

The economic impact of new technology has two major dimensions: new technology is a major contributer to inflation; and opportunity costs associated with new technology involve vast expenditures, that if used more efficiently or for other purposes would yield greater public benefit.

In recent years, 50 percent of the cost of hospital care was attributed to medical technology. The capital costs receive the most attention, especially the big dollar items such as CAT scanners. However, it is the operating support costs that usually constitute the most expensive component of new technology. Staff must be hired and receive specialized training to operate new equipment. In order to justify capital and staff expenditures, the new technology is "marketed" and too frequently overused. New technology is used and public and private insurance pays the bills, without question. One encouraging development is that Blue Cross recently announced that it will no longer routinely reimburse hospitals for all diagnostic procedures, unless justified.

The disproportionate amount of money used to support new technology has raised serious questions about resource allocation. According to Warner,[5] if funds expended for Medicare were used for alternate purposes, the 3.3 million aged poor could be raised above the poverty level, or rent could be paid that would allow the 2.2 million aged living in substandard housing to move into standard housing.

There are also questions about the amount of the health care dollar used for high technology that might be better used for more basic, less expensive services. In many respects, the health care we receive today is shaped by medical technology, rather than need. It is estimated that the excess supply and use of medical technology in New York State alone costs well over $100 million dollars a year. Overemphasizing sophisticated technology diminishes the importance of basic health care services. As the supply of primary and preventive services is shrinking in New York City, hospitals continue to purchase new equipment and open new facilities to develop highly specialized services. If these funds could instead be used to provide basic primary care services where needed, it is likely that health status would improve, and it would be possible to eliminate federally designated medically underserved areas in New York State. Indeed, the cost of supporting our fancy for the exotic in medical technology is quite high, in fiscal and human terms.

A Public Interest Approach to Medical Technology

Finite resources require that we make choices on how to best spend the health care dollar. "Scientific merit" should not place the development and dissemination of new technology above public accountability when choices have to be made.

The impact of new medical technology must be evaluated before it is disseminated. A publicly accountable, systematic, and comprehensive framework for assessing the broad implications of new technology is needed before it is introduced into the health care delivery system. A comprehensive assessment should go beyond evaluating safety and efficacy. The U.S. Congress, Office of Technology Assessment (OTA), suggested that discussions of such assessment should answer the following questions:

1. What medical problems is new technology designed to address? Does it prevent or cure, or does it provide a more limited or halfway remedy?
2. How many people are served and what are potential outcomes (also, side effects)?
3. What is anticipated use and potential for its use?
4. What are costs to the individual patient and the economy?
5. What are alternatives for same illness?
6. What are the choices regarding alternative use of funds?
7. What is the impact on the health care delivery system?[6]

An early alert system must be developed at the federal, state, and local levels in order to assess and plan prior to dissemination of new technology.

At the federal level, there are many agencies that perform technology assessment (from lesser to greater degrees). The most effective assessment machinery is in the Food and Drug Administration, which has had long-standing assessment and regulatory authority over prescription drugs, and in 1976 was given expanded authority over medical devices. Other federal agencies (e.g., NIH, National Center for Health Services Research, Office of Health Practice Assessment, Health Standards and Quality Bureau) perform different aspects of assessment (e.g., safety, efficacy, cost-effectiveness).

Although different government agencies do perform elements of technology assessment, these elements are not linked together and do not follow each other logically; a formal or well-coordinated system for developing and disseminating needed information for decision making does not exist. The Office of Technology Assessment identified the following shortcomings in the assessment process:

> Assessment is fragmented, lacking a well coordinated overall system.
>
> No formal mechanism exists for identifying technologies to be studied.
>
> Inadequate attention and funding to various steps in assessment.
>
> The federal government has not given sufficient priority to disseminating information.[7]

A step towards correcting these problems would be establishing a federal authority over all health research activity for identifying, assessing, and coordinating the development of new technology. The authority should not be placed in an agency that directly supports research and development activity (e.g., NIH) because of the potential for conflict of interest.

The National Center for Health Care Technology, created by the Health Services Research, Health Statistics and Health Care Technology Act of 1978, would appear to be a suitable locus for carrying out these assessment and coordination functions.

The National Center for Health Care Technology has two major missions:

1. It should stimulate increased scrutiny of new and existing health care technologies to insure that their safety; efficacy; cost-effectivensss; and social, ethical, and economic impacts are more completely explored.
2. Encourage the rapid dissemination of newly developed health care technologies which have proved their worth in terms of safety, efficacy, and cost-effectiveness.[8]

In addition to the creation of the National Center for Health Care Technology, the new law provides for the following:

1. Creation of a National Council for the Evaluation of Medical Technology to develop and disseminate standards, norms and criteria concerning the utilization of specific technologies. The "Council" would be strengthened if it were in some fashion formally connected with the National Council on Health Planning and Development and the National Professional Standards Review Council.
2. Funding support for the creation of public and private nonprofit centers to assess health care technology.
3. Authorizes the "Center" to make recommendations concerning administration and reimbursement policies in Medicaid and Medicare in regard to new technology.[9]

At the time of this writing, it would be premature to attempt to assess the extent to which HEW has fulfilled its reponsibilities under this new law.

The Health Planning Law (P.L. 93-641) requires that state and local planning agencies determine that "need" exists prior to approval of new capital expense projects. "Appropriateness review," (which, to date, has not been defined adequately for implementation) holds out the *potential* for planning agencies to review existing programs and services, with similar criteria, and the *potential* for approving or denying the continuation of existing programs. The National Council for the Evaluation of Medical Technology should issue guidelines (based on standards, norms, and criteria) that would in term be adapted by state and local planning agencies for regional application.

The State Health Planning and Development Agency (SHPDA) and the local HSA have specific decision-making responsibilities. In the past, the decisions were not made, or made too late, or made in a vacuum without sufficient data. With adequate information, the SHPDA, in consultation with the HSAs should be responsible for developing a plan for dissemination of new technologies based on the needs assessment framework suggested by OTA. Given the high cost that is often associated with new technology and the usual pressure of all 300,000 physicians and 7,000 hospitals in the nation desiring to "acquire" the latest technology, SHPDAs and HSAs should place special emphasis on avoiding duplication, understanding the costs involved, with particular attention to alternative needs (e.g., primary care) to which limited health care dollars may be applied. Special attention should be given to ensure a fair distribution of new technology that would improve population access. This is particularly important at the initial stages of dissemination.

These plans should be developed in formal consultation with Professional Standards Review Organizations (PSROs). PSRO linkage not only actively involves the participation of informed provider groups concerned with the effects of different types of medical intervention, but it offers the potential of acquiring data on the effects of certain new technologies that would be useful for future decision making.

Once a state plan is established, state Certificate-of-Need regulations should be issued for the dissemination of the new technology, and should include reimbursement penalties for unapproved use of new technology. The HSAs local Health Systems Plan (HSP) should include a plan for local distribution of new technology, based on state criteria. If this can be achieved on the basis of need and adequate information, new technology can be used to serve the public interest by fulfilling the priority goals and objectives of the HSP.

To succeed, a coordinated federal, state, and local early identification, assessment, and dissemination strategy must begin at the earliest stage of research and development before the fact. If it begins during the dissemination stage, it is after the fact, and too late. The choice is simple and complex. Will new technology be shaped to meet the public interest, or will the public interest be shaped to accommodate new technology?

References

1. Office of Technology Assessment. *Assessing the efficacy and safety of medical technologies.* U.S. Congress, Washington, D.C.: U.S. Govt. Printing Office, September, 1978, p. XII.
2. Bennett, I. L., Jr. Technology as a shaping force, in J. H. Knowles (Ed.) *Doing better and feeling worse.* New York: Norton, 1977.
3. Thomas, L. *Aspects of biomedical science policy: an occasional paper.* Washington, D.C.: Institute of Medicine, 1972.
4. Geiger, H. J. Who shall live by V. R. Fuchs. *New York Times Book Review,* March 2, 1975.
5. Warner, K. E. Effects of hospital cost containment on the development and use of medical technology. *Milbank Memorial Fund Quarterly,* 1978, *56*(2), 187–211.

6. Office of Technology Assessment. *Development of medical technology: Opportunities for assessment.* U.S. Congress, Washington, D.C.: U.S. Govt Printing Office, 1976.
7. Office of Technology Assessment, September 1978 Ibid.
8. U.S. House of Representatives. *Conference report: Health services research, health statistics and health care technology act of 1978.* Report No. 95-1783, 95th Congress, Second Session, October 13, 1978.
9. Ibid.

Chapter 12

THE SPIRALING COSTS OF MEDICAL CARE: IS MEDICAL TECHNOLOGY THE VILLAIN?

Herbert Harvey Hyman

A few years ago, a poll was taken of New York City residents in which they were asked to rank the major problems that concerned them. Only 5 percent of those surveyed cited health care issues as major problems. Crime, dirty streets, unemployment, and noise ran well ahead of health-related problems. Things have changed since that early 1970 poll. The cost of medical care has come to concern more and more people. Hospital costs have become the number one inflation-related concern of the Carter administration. We hear about the 1000 percent increase in the cost of a day of hospital care over the last 25 years; the 100 percent increase of the last five years.[1] We hear about the 9 percent cap President Carter wants placed on the total increases in health care for 1979/1980. We hear about union workers wanting more take home pay and fewer deductions taken out for their medical care fringe benefits. The new radiology equipment, the CAT scanners, cost $400,000 to $600,000 to purchase and half that amount again to maintain them annually. We hear about the great emphasis Health Sys-

Reprinted from *Connecticut Medicine*, 1979. Used with permission.

tems Agencies place on cost containment and the standards promulgated recently by HEW to limit the number of beds, expensive medical procedures, and equipment. And we all hear from our neighbors about the out-of-pocket costs they must pay for drugs, physician fees, and dental care. In brief, the high cost of medical care is beginning to have its impact on an ever widening circle of Americans and they are letting their representatives in Congress know about it.

Although all of the components of medical care are rising in cost, it is the cost of hospitalization that is going up most quickly. And it is usually the hospital which has the financial capacity to purchase expensive equipment and hire highly paid physicians and technologists to operate this equipment. Consequently, a brief examination of the trends in hospital costs is essential. Hospital costs are traditionally divided into two segments, labor and nonlabor. In 1955, labor amounted to 62 percent of the costs of a hospital day of care. Nonlabor (which includes medical technology) costs were 38 percent; by 1969, labor component was reduced to 59 percent; by 1975, it was reduced to 53 percent.[2] In brief, the medical equipment and other nonlabor costs were rising far more rapidly than the costs of labor. This in spite of the fact that hospital workers' wages increased more quickly than the average wage of all other industries. Thus, at first glance we can state that medical technology and our love affair with it may well be the villain in the rapidly escalating costs of medical care. But, before we jump to that conclusion it is necessary to examine the historical background that led to this marriage between the hospital and medical technology.

How It Happened

Starting with the Great Depression and continuing into the end of World War II, there were either no funds to build new hospitals or there were no construction materials available to build them because the war effort held first claim. Thus, for a period of almost 20 years little or no building of new hospitals took place. Following World War II and continuing for several years into the early 1950s, there was a huge backlog of consumer demands for public works, particularly roads and sewer systems, and for public necessities such as schools and hospitals. In this period of expanding the nation's store of capital goods and of refurbishing industrial plants and buildings of the United States, three significant occurrences, two in the health field and one in foreign relations, profoundly affected and set the course for our love affair with technology.

First, the Hill-Burton Act was passed in 1946 to assist small communities and especially rural communities to build community hospitals and facilities that would attract physicians. In the next 30 years, some $15 billion dollars were spent on hospital expansion with the federal government supplying one-third of it under matching formulas.[3] These buildings required the latest equipment commensurate with the level of modern treatment they intended to provide to patients. Thus, this bill was a major impetus for the hospital equipment industry and hospital suppliers to develop newer, more efficient, and consequently more costly ways of treating patients.

Second, the governmentally funded National Institutes of Health, which began in 1938 with the establishment of the National Cancer Institute, experienced major growth from the 1950s until the mid-1970s when a brake was put on increasing their expenditures. The original institute concerned with cancer grew to include 10 different disease entities at a cost of more than $14 billion dollars over the last 20 years. This huge sum of money was spent solely on medical research with the great medical schools of New York City alone receiving about 10 percent of the funds. This emphasis on medical research in our medical schools and teaching hospitals fostered the specialties and superspecialties with which we are so familiar today. Federal money spawned a nation of medical scientists for whom the practice of medicine was secondary to research and teaching.

Newly educated physicians learned about the marvels of the new technology that were issuing from the medical suppliers as well as about the research undertaken by their colleagues in medical institutions.

Third, an international space race was touched off by Russia's sending a satellite into orbit. This coup was followed by a declaration of President Kennedy and Congress to beat the Russians to the moon. Billions of dollars were poured into this effort and led to the application of existing technology to space vehicles and to the development of new technology to monitor the astronauts' health. Some of these new inventions were directly applicable to advancing the medical technologies used in treating patients. Laser beams were applied to the treatment of cancer, and computers and electronic equipment led to the development of the new CAT scanners.

While there are many other factors that led to the fantastic growth of technology and its application to diagnosis and treatment of patients, these three appear to be the most significant. Directly and indirectly they spurred the initial increase in medical technology and research and helped to maintain its growth.

American Public Demands the Best

The emphasis placed on medical technology also has been blessed by the average American. Progress in the United States has always been associated with material advances and the invention of new gadgets. Americans quickly grow tired of their possessions and demand new fashions, fixtures, equipment, utensils, accessories, homes, cars, and entertainment. This demand for the latest carries over to the physician's office and to the hospital. Americans are aware of the new buildings, the new equipment, and the increased number of staff when they enter a hospital. And they are willing to pay for these improvements.

It is the way they pay for these costs, however, that make them immune to the real costs of service. They have sacrificed higher take-home pay for increased medical benefits. Because employees always received a real pay increase along with an increase in their fringe benefits, they have not looked upon the higher costs of fringe benefits as a sacrifice. Second, the insurance industry's development of the major medical concept has further reduced the strain on a person's savings in the event of a catastrophic illness. The combination of the insurers' paying the first dollar costs for 90 to 95 percent of a short hospital stay plus major medical coverage for serious or prolonged illness has cushioned the average American from the brunt of major health care expenses. When one adds to the insurance that substitutes for lost pay due to illness, the average American is almost immune from paying or feeling the economic impact of high cost hospital expenses. This fact is borne out in a study of the net cost of hospital care to the consumer over a 25-year period.[4] That study clearly shows that the amount a person paid out of his own pocket in 1950 for a day of hospital care was $7.75 or 50 percent of the total cost (the rest being paid by government or medical insurance). By 1975, the patient paid $18.03, but insurance paid $133 of the average $151 per day cost. This 1975 out-of-pocket cost represents only 12 percent of the hospital bill, a great reduction from 1950. Even more amazing is that the part of his spendable income that was spent on hospital care hardly changed at all between 1950 and 1975. In 1950, the average worker spent 19 percent of his or her income on hospital care and in 1975, it had increased to only 22 percent. In sum, the worker hardly feels the dramatically increased cost of hospital care as a special economic burden.

Low economic cost to the worker may not be the most important factor associated with his or her acceptance of rapidly increasing hospital costs. Regardless of differences in income and expenditure patterns, the average American emulates the rich. By sacrificing small amounts of take home pay for medical insurance benefits, Americans can feel on a par with the wealthy when it comes to obtaining medical treatment in the hospital. Having paid their dues with medical insurance, they demand the best care. If they feel cheated or neglected in their efforts to secure this high quality care, they are quick to strike back at the physician or hospital with costly malpractice suits, or vociferous complaints about the service received from the medical provider. The public wants to be treated the way providers treat the wealthy. This means the use of expensive medical procedures, regardless of cost.

Probably the most important factor, however, is the average American's great faith in the capacity of American technology to cure illness. Consumers want medical science and the technologic equipment developed by it to extend their lives, to improve their capacity to function in a relatively normal manner, and to reduce or eliminate pain associated with illness or disease. And they want this at little or no economic, psychological, physical, or social cost to themselves. The patient wants a personal miracle through the use of our latest technologic advances. This belief in the miracles of medical science is strong in Americans in spite of the evidence to the contrary. Colman[5] has stated:

> Positive health can be achieved only through intelligent effort on the part of each individual. Absent that effort, health professionals can only insulate the individual from the more catastrophic results of his ignorance, self-indulgence, or lack of motivation.

Victor Fuchs[6] seriously doubts that the spread of medical technology has contributed much to the health of Americans or that its future expansion would make much difference. However, the facts are not as important to the consumer as his own perceptions of what medical technology can do for him or her in time of serious illness.

Physician Education

In 1972, there were 320,000 active physicians. Of these, 250,000 or 78 percent worked in a specialty area. Since 1954, there has been a steady increase in medical schools, from 81 in

1954, to 108 in 1971. Along with this increase has been a larger number of graduates from 7,000 in 1954 to 10,000 in 1972.[7] In 1972, 87 percent of the residency positions available were filled. Only one category deviated greatly from that average. Only 60 percent of the general practice residency positions were filled.[8] Surgery, internal medicine, pediatrics, radiology, and so forth had little difficulty filling the great majority of their positions. What do these isolated bits of data tell us?

First, that American doctors are a product of their society. Since society places a higher premium on specialization, the great majority of medical students specialize when they enter practice. Specialization is related intimately to learning how to master and use the medical technology associated with that specialty. Therefore, both in medical school and later in their residencies, our future physicians become familiar with and comfortable in handling ever more exotic equipment. Many of them become fascinated enough by this technology that they are readily lured into medical research using the billions of dollars poured into the medical schools and teaching hospitals by the National Institutes of Health and large private foundations. Articles relating their discoveries pour forth by the thousands each year. The best practitioners and researchers become much sought after as faculty members and chiefs of staff in their specialty. Government agencies and foundations provide more research funds to these eminent men of medical science. Suppliers court their favor and sell them the latest equipment to use in their experiments or their treatment of patients. In turn, these physicians teach their students the complexities of diagnostic and treatment equipment. Upon graduation and after fulfilling their residency requirements, these newly indoctrinated physicians desire to practice only where they have access to this technology. It gives them power, influence, status, and promise of high income. Therefore, it is not surprising that they gravitate to the urban and suburban centers where most of the large, prestigious medical schools and teaching hospitals are located. Community hospitals and rural clinics are just too small and isolated from the medicine they learned and the colleagues with whom they desire to be associated. And the American public is satisfied for them to be located in the populous urban centers and suburbs where most live. The tendency of the health care system to emphasize these more sophisticated elements of diagnosis and treatment has been referred to as the "technologic imperative."[9] Compared to the mundane practice of family medicine with its treatment of common, usually self-curing ailments, a medical practice associated with complex equipment and elaborate facilities in a prestige hospital is considered the only true way to practice medicine. As long as the American public perceives that the prolongation of life is linked inextricably to treatment by medical specialists manning a battery of sophisticated machines, physicians will be trained and educated to satisfy this need.

Explosion in Number of Medical Technologists

In spite of the physicians' medical education, they could not possibly operate and maintain this sophisticated equipment without a whole array of allied medical support technologists. Just as there has been an expansion of medical schools so too have there been the birth and expansion of many training programs for the technologist. A list of these changes will illustrate the growth of these numerous subspecialty technical positions.

Practical nurse training: 16,500 graduates in 1960 and 44,000 in 1972.

Physical therapists: 682 graduates in 1961 and 2300 in 1973.

Radiologic technology: 2300 graduates in 1962 and 6300 in 1973.

Musical Therapists: 18 graduates in 1962 and 140 in 1973.

Speech Pathology/Audiology: 2250 graduates in 1961 and 9200 in 1973.

Medical Record Administrators: 137 in 1960 and 263 in 1972.

Health and Vital Statistics: 15,600 graduates in 1961 and 30,700 in 1971.

Public Health Nutrition: 33 graduates in 1960 and 123 in 1972.

Dental Hygienists: 1200 graduates in 1962 and 3400 in 1972.

Cytotechnologists: 290 graduates in 1963 and 427 in 1971.

In addition, there are programs in biomedical engineering; automatic data processing; economic research in health, orthotic, and prosthetic technology; and specialized rehabilitation services.[10] A quick examination of the statistics shows that there has been from two- to tenfold or more increase in graduates produced by these various degree programs. The physician, who commands these growing resources of support specialists, requires a first hand knowledge of what they do so he can properly supervise their work and order tests required for patients. As of 1974, the National Center for Health Statistics identified almost 100 specialties in the medical care field and the number keeps growing. Over 4.5 million workers are connected with these specialties, most of which did not exist 25 years ago. They are a product of our demand for high quality care based on specialization. Of course, the technologists become a force in their own right and are making their demands on the health care system for recognition and status. Any thought of changing the medical emphasis on technology would require dealing with this formidable force that has grown so rapidly in the last 15 years. While the explosion may have abated somewhat the last few years, its major growth has already occurred. Almost all such positions are wedded to sophisticated medical technologies and equipment.

The Others: Hospital Trustees, Administrators, and Insurance Companies

The American competitive urge also infects the board rooms and the hospital administrator's office. Striving to be numer one is infectious, especially if it is relatively costless. To lure physicians trained at the best medical schools, the hospital administrators must supply the space, equipment, and ancillary personnel to meet the physician's needs. The board of trustees, usually business-oriented leaders themselves, are as much in tune with this competitive spirit as are their administrators. As long as most, if not all, of the costs of medical technology are borne by governmental, nonprofit, and commercial health insurers, then it becomes even more attractive to purchase the very best. Since the added costs of most of these new medical inventions are buried in the increased per diem costs, the incremental increases do not seem to point to any one medical technology as the cause of the increase in hospital care. No one asks, or is even concerned with answering, whether the new equipment makes a difference to the life, comfort, and well-being of the patients or their families. The fact is that no one really knows the answer to such a question. For an individual patient, it is possible to offer a specific answer. How applicable that answer is to others undergoing the same treatment is unknown. Administrators and their boards are satisfied with their hospital additions, as are the physicians with the latest knowledge learned at the best medical schools and the equipment supplied for their use. The hospital's competitive position is maintained or improved.

Thus, there are a number of interacting, but autonomous, forces at work that encourage the use, experimentation, and continued diffusion of medical technology in our hospitals, clinics, and physicians' offices. There has been little reason to raise questions up to now about this trend and more reason to support it.

Who Pays for the New Technology?

There are four major sources of funds for meeting health expenditures: public financing, private/nonprofit insurance companies, out-of-pocket expenses, and private philanthropy. All four sources directly and indirectly pay for the costs of introducing medical technology into the mainstream of health care. As one researcher[11] discovered, "the great majority of new technologies are introduced within the current reimbursement system." These reimbursement measures include Medicaid, Medicare, Blue Cross, and commercial insurance companies. This is done with the concurrence of the American public through support of Congressional actions respecting governmental medical programs and in the private sector through the support of increased health benefits negotiated in union contracts. Within recent years, workers demanded higher take home pay and Congress and the executive branch became concerned with the escalating costs of health care. Now greater attention is paid health costs and particularly those associated with hospital care.

However, new costly experimental programs are not always reimbursed under third-party contracts. Nonetheless, sources of funding are still quite available for experimentation. The largest source of these funds emanates from the national health institutes, going primarily to the large medical schools, teaching hospitals, and specialized hospitals and laboratories, including universities. Supplementing these funds are special philanthropic grants from wealthy individuals or their endowed foundations. In many instances, even this new experimentation becomes accepted as normal and routine once findings have been reported in conferences and professional journals. As the individual medical technology spreads as accepted practice, often while it is still in its developmental stage, it becomes a part of the per diem operating costs that are subject to reimbursement from health care insurers. How it occurs that a new medical technology is transformed from excepted, nonreimbursable costs in some institutions to part of the per diem charges in other institutions where it has been adopted is still not well understood. Nevertheless, until very recently, the increased costs were sanctioned and eventually accepted as part of the hospital's cost of providing service.

Economic Outcomes

An examination of the data available indicates that a number of factors have been responsible for the rapid increase of hospital costs. Among these are:

1. Increase in nonpayroll expenses
2. Increase in payroll expenses
3. Inflation
4. Increase due to greater utilization, especially of short-stay acute care beds
5. Population growth

Of these five factors, the increases in payroll and nonpayroll expenses accounted for almost 70 percent of the increase in costs between 1965 and 1973.[12] Adding inflation to these two factors, they accounted for 90 percent. The two smallest factors are increased use and population growth. Increased costs due to payroll expenses are explained by a number of factors. The number of personnel per patient rose from 2.26 in 1960 to 3.15 in 1973, a 72 percent increase. With the swift dissemination of expensive and complex medical technology, the type of staff hired to operate these machines and equipment is more costly than heretofore. I noted earlier the rapid increase of a number of ancillary well-trained staff to meet the operation and maintenance needs of the hospitals. Furthermore, this has been a period of rapid wage increases. Hospital staff traditionally were one of the lowest paid industries prior to the 1960s. With the advent of Medicaid and Medicare and the general acceptance by third-party insurers of rapidly increasing per diem rates, additional costs were passed onto the consumer. Hospital workers not only caught up to the general earning levels of the average American worker, but passed them and are slowly widening the gap in their favor.[13] There are more highly trained and better paid hospital personnel in 1975 than in 1965.

Nonpayroll costs rose even more rapidly than labor costs. From 1955 to 1975, labor costs rose by 9 percent per year, whereas nonpayroll costs increased by 11 percent.[14] A recent study of 24 medical technologic innovations shows that they had differential impacts on several hospital indicators from 1960 to 1972.[15] There was a decrease in the number of hospital days in 14 diseases treated by these innovations, some dramatically lower. For example, there were 950,000 fewer patient days for nephrotic syndrome in 1972 than in 1960; 365,000 fewer days for duodenal ulcers in the same time period; and 80,000 fewer days for acute nephritis. On the other hand, 12 of the diseases witnessed increased hospital days, the most dramatic being arteriosclerosis by 1 million days, cataracts by 725,000 days, and osteoarthritis by 661,000 days. The same is true for hospital discharges per 100,000 persons and mean length of stay. There were increases and decreases due to the innovations. However, with respect to physician visits and prescription drug use, there were dramatic increases as ongoing, follow-up treatment was generally required to maintain close scrutiny of the patients who had been treated with these medical innovations. This study further shows that for 16 surgical-medical innovations used in 1970, the return on costs of 21 million dollars expended by the National Institutes of Health for biomedical research resulted in an estimated $2.8 billion dollars of benefits as measured by reduced mortality and a higher rate of returning to productive work. This is a cost benefit ratio of 135:1. While this is truly an astounding cost-benefit ratio, the study notes that if all the costs, including training grants, continuing research, and constructions costs were added, the cost-benefit ratio would be reduced to 1.7:1, still a positive finding. While there was a rise in medical technology costs, the cost-benefit ratio indicated that there was an economic pay-off in the use of such innovations.

At the same time, these benefits are costing the consumer, in net costs relative to the prices of other goods and services, less in 1974 than they did in 1950. Measured by the prices of 1967, the net cost of a day of hospital care was $10.75 in 1950 and only $10.23 in 1974.[16] This truly remarkable fact helps to account for the consumer's relative lack of interest in the rise in the costs of health care. For a lower net cost, consumers receive better care in new facilities which use the latest medical technology. How could there be a better bargain?

The Cycle

When one takes these various factors into account, it seems that the medical industry, and hospitals in particular, are simply being responsive to the demands of the consumer. Finding hospital care a bargain compared to other goods and services, the consumer demands more and better services. Physicians oblige by putting pressure on the hospitals to supply the newest medical innovations. Looked at in this way, there is really no one villain in the crowd, not the physician, nor the hospital, nor the consumers. All are part of a cycle, each putting pressure on the other to have their own best interests met. Because the cycle interrelates so well, it becomes difficult to know where to intervene at all. Yet, why is there a growing chorus at this time to hold down the escalating costs of hospital care, and medical technology in particular?

THE REACTION: WHY IT'S COMING NOW

Reactions to medical costs emanate from two sources, national and international affairs affecting the American economy and the desire to brake the costs of care by some consumer elements exerting their influence on Congress and the President. First, let us examine some of the forces at work on the national and international levels. Three forces have been at work and are now profoundly influencing the American economy. First, the oil embargo and the resulting energy crisis dramatically escalated the costs of gas and oil. It has also increased our dependence on Arab and other oil-producing nations. Forced to pay higher costs for energy, the average American has less money to spend for other needs.

The oil embargo triggered off a general recession mingled with inflation. Inflationary costs are wiping out any gains made by American workers and their unions. Union members repeatedly rejected contracts negotiated by their leaders. Not only are they concerned about job security, but they want more take-home pay to offset galloping inflation. When the union negotiators cast about for ways to achieve this, one component of the wage package that came to their attention was the amount of money allocated for health care insurance. They were targeting health care benefits because they were so visible and costly. Unions and the corporations are beginning to ask questions about these costs. There is even consideration on the part of some of our leading corporations to develop their own insurance plans in an effort to reduce the price of health care premiums. Once cozy relationships existed among many of these same corporate leaders as members of the hospital boards of leading institutions. Now, this relationship is putting a strain on them as they witness how their hospital decisions influence their own costs of doing business. Consequently, they give closer scrutiny to these decisions. Unions are moving simultaneously in two potentially opposite directions with respect to health care costs. On one hand, they are pressing for the control of national health care costs; on the other hand, they are pressing for a national health insurance plan that will raise costs, but shift the expenditures from the bargaining table to the government. Union members are becoming active in health planning agencies in order to press for those components of the plans that will reduce overall health costs, with special emphasis on making the hospitals more efficient in their use of facilities and equipment. In this regard, there is a focus on medical technology and efforts to prevent its diffusion and unnecessary duplication.

A third force reacting to higher costs of health care is the public's general lack of confidence in the efficiency of federal, state, and local government itself. This trend was evident in the issues raised during the last presidential campaign and in the current symptoms of a taxpayer's revolt, embodied in numerous defeats of local education budgets and in the passage of California's Proposition 13. While many areas of high government expenditures are being examined, health care is one of the areas coming under close scrutiny. People are particularly upset with sporadic reports citing higher than expected income for physicians under Medicaid payments, the shuffling of patients for profit, the charging for services never rendered, and the provision of services for which there is no medical problem. Pressure has been brought to bear to put a ceiling on physician payments for services rendered as well as holding the line on publicly controlled expenditures in the operation of hospitals. In New York City, 6000 to 7000 beds were closed in the municipal system in the past decade. This action would have been welcomed as an effort to reduce the number of excess beds except for the fact that an almost equal number of beds have been opened in the same period of time in the voluntary private sector. All that this does is raise questions by the public and by the citizens' bodies that monitor the health care field about the credibility of their leaders and their apparent abuse of the public trust. Indeed, Roemer's[17] principle says that if there are empty beds they will be filled, whether services are truly needed or not.

Thus, these three external forces have upset the general American economy and brought concern to workers about their own job security and ability to earn enough income to maintain their standard of living. While there is general concern about government in general, there is particular emphasis on reducing the costs of health care. These costs are more and more being perceived as eating away at the take home pay needed by the average worker.

Internally, there has been a mixed picture of how valuable the use of medical technology really is. There are those who raise questions about whether medical technology makes any difference at all in health outcomes.[18] There has been no appreciable reduction in either the morbidity or mortality rates in spite of the heavy investment in these innovations. Some have stated that the emphasis in NIH allocation of funds is misplaced. It is pointed out that "mental illness, which ranks third in cause of days of hospitalization and fourth in cause of limitation of activity, received only 6 percent of these outlays. Only 7 percent went for research on arthritis, metabolic and digestive problems, which together are the leading causes of days of hospitalization."[19] Furthermore, some noted that the emphasis on research has deemphasized the treatment of the more common diseases and illnesses in community hospitals. As one investigator stated, "medical intervention has a significant effect on outcome in only a small fraction of the cases seen by the average physician."[20] Most illnesses are either self-limiting and require no medical treatment, or are chronic and incurable. Chronic illnesses require a physician to emphasize the "caring" rather than the "curing," an art that is rapidly being lost in the medical schools' love affair with technology.

On the other hand, there are those who point out the benefits of medical technology. A favorable cost-benefit ratio motivates the expenditure of millions on technology. For example, the CAT scanner reduces both hospitalization costs and pain to patients treated with pneumoencephalography. [21] Another researcher noted that in 1970 alone, the application of 17 different medical inventions used in surgery for various diseases prevented the deaths of 65,000 persons had the technology not been used.[22] Furthermore, for nine different disease categories such as peptic ulcer, heart conditions, and hearing impairments, there were significant improvements between the years 1961 and 1969 on three health indicators. With respect to limitation of a person's activity, there was improvement in eight of the nine disease categories. In six of the nine categories, there were fewer work days lost; and in all nine categories, there were fewer cases of bed-ridden disability.[23] However, this same researcher noted that the prevalence of the diseases in the population increased, in some cases dramatically, during the eight years. For example, the cases per 1,000 population show more than a 50 percent increase in prevalance of heart conditions, hypertension without heart involvement, arthritis and rheumatism, and visual and hearing impairments. These statistics provide ammunition to those opposed to the expansion and almost exclusive emphasis on medical technology. It does little to prevent people from getting ill, even though it may be of benefit to them once they do. Too much of our resources are going to treating illnesses and not enough to preventing them. Thus, while there are pro- and antimedical technology forces, each is looking at the situation from its own perspective. It really comes down to a philosophy of medicine. Do we put most of our emphasis on prevention and public health, or on diagnosis and treatment and medical care? Thus far, the medical care forces have won the battle hands down.

Yet, the "anti"-forces are not idle. Labor spokesmen, civic organizations, and numerous minority groups who feel they are being squeezed out of the medical care system have been putting pressure on their congressional representatives and leaders to take measures to halt the escalation of medical care costs. Congress responded in two directions, passing legislation to reduce medical costs and to plan a more rational system.

With respect to cost containment measures, Congress made efforts to reduce the cost of care by encouraging the use of physician and dental assistants. While health care assistants provided more care, especially in low-income communities, it is not certain whether medical care costs have been lowered by their addition. President Nixon gave a significant boost to using lower cost ambulatory care facilities by pressing for the expansion of the nascent prepaid health maintenance organization movement with planning and construction dollars. After a number of slow starts, there was a recent upsurge in the development of HMOs around the country. Yet, it is doubted that HMOs will make a significant impact in weaning patients away from their relationships with private physicians. In addition, Congress has been trying to hold the line on expenditures for medical education, NIH medical technology research, hospital construction, and Medicaid and Medicare. While there is a renewed interest in national health insurance, the prevailing mood in Congress and the executive branch is to hold off such a far-reaching and potentially costly measure until the costs of health care have been brought under control. Finally, regulatory measures such as Certificate-Of-Need for hospital construction and renovation, prospective rate setting to maintain a ceiling on the annual costs of operating a hospital, and medical audits and reviews of utilization of hospital, long-term care, and ambulatory services are further efforts by Congress to brake the rising costs of medical care. However, in spite of the passage of all these measures in the last 5 to 10 years, there has been no appreciable slowing in the increased costs of such care.

This finally led Congress to try a new tack. If health plans can actually be developed for each service region in the United States, HEW might be in a position to assess what the real problems in the system are and what alternatives might be attempted to provide improved care at lower cost. At the same time, HEW thought that linking planning to regulation might have an impact on rising costs that neither by itself is able to accomplish.

HEALTH PLANNING AND REGULATION: P.L. 93-641

The Health Planning and Resources Development Act of 1974 was passed by Congress for the express purposes of 1) containing the cost of medical care, and 2) improving the quality of care. Both of these goals are laudable. However, they are potentially in conflict. How is it possible to raise the quality of care without costing more money? Congressional leaders, working in tandem with HEW officials, identified 10 priorities in the Act. If carried out to their maximum, these priorities would achieve both goals. Section 1502 of the Act identifies these 10 priorities. Their major thrust is on improving efficiency in the use of medical services. They call for such changes as:

- Integrating services where possible
- Regionalizing services so that continuity of care is maintained
- Using lower cost services such as physician assistants
- Reducing the unnecessary lengths of hospital stay by utilization review
- Emphasizing lower cost services such as HMOs, home health and ambulatory surgicenters

Through these combined measures and others like them, the waste would be washed out of the medical care system. With the savings accrued from these sources, the Health Systems Agencies would be able to identify priorities for providing better services to underserved populations. Out of money saved through reduction in waste and duplication of services, the potential conflict between the goals of cost containment and quality would be merged into a positive accommodation. That is the theory. What is the reality as it has been played out up to this point?

Health Planning

HSAs are required by law to develop five-year and one-year implementation plans within two years of their creation as planning agencies. By and large, almost all the HSAs have developed such plans. They are huge documents ranging from 300 pages to well over 1000 pages in length, not including even larger appendices that have accompanied most of the plans in Region II, which includes New York and New Jersey. As a professor interested in planning, I have examined these plans and found that they more or less conform to guidelines set forth by HEW. While it is not possible to speak about regionwide priorities, one of the main components to which the goals speak are the regionalization of one or more specialized medical services. These include services requiring high costs of equipment, space, and personnel such as burn centers, CAT scanners, automated laboratory equipment, diagnostic radiology, renal dialysis, and open heart surgery.

All of these services will cost more than the $150,000 minimum set by HEW guidelines, requiring review by HSAs and state regulatory bodies to determine whether they are needed. That is a commendable function of the HSAs and the state. However, in the past, the regulatory function of the HSAs (determining whether an expensive piece of medical equipment is needed) has often been in conflict with their planning function. With the development of plans, goals should speak to the priority or importance of the region's acquiring such equipment, how many units are necessary, where they ought to be located, and for whose benefit they are used. Unfortunately, there has been an inconsistency between the state guidelines for these specialized medical technologies and the criteria used by the HSAs within the states. HSAs themselves developed widely differing criteria and standards for the review of such projects. One researcher counted 32 state agencies and/or HSAs that have developed guidelines and criteria used in their review of CAT scanners. On only 4 of the 10 criteria identified (requirement of full-time neurosurgeon, neurologist, and radiologist and regionalization of the scanners to insure both availability and access) was there anything approaching consensus on whether to approve the CAT scanner proposal or not.[24] If there is this degree of difference over the proper criteria to review CAT scanners, which have received so much attention in the past three years, there is likely to be even more confusion about how to review the other specilized medical technologies.

Few of the 13 plans developed by Region II HSAs state where specialized services rank in their priorities (most HSAs have not stated what any of their priorities are). Plans more usually contain a general statement that studies should be undertaken to determine how such services can be regionalized. In some instances, as in the Bergen-Passaic Plan (New Jersey), the specialized services and their locations were identified. This is more the exception than the rule. To put some rationality into the HSAs' thinking, HEW developed minimum guidelines for 11 components of health care, 9 of which deal with specialized medical technology.[25] For example, no CAT scanner should be approved unless it can show evidence of producing a minimum of 2500 scans a year. Radiation therapy for cancer cases requires approval for those proposals where at least 7500 treatments per year will be rendered and where there is a likelihood that 450 new cancer cases will be found. At least 200 procedures are the minimum number required before approval can be given for an open heart surgical unit. These represent a beginning, but they still offer much room for the HSAs and state agencies to develop further criteria to determine need.

Thus, while there is some confusion about how to link the planning and regulatory functions, increasing attention is being given to medical technology because of the prominent role it plays in the costs of providing hospital services.

Rate Setting

In addition to planning and regulation, the Act calls for developing rate-setting experiments in seven states. The purpose of the experiments is to apply different models for determining the funds required by a hospital for the following year and holding it to that level of expenditure. This is called prospective rate setting. By setting such a ceiling, the burden is then shifted to the medical facility to find ways to make its own institution more efficient rather than having this task imposed by the state. The concern about prospective reimbursement is that an institution with unusual expenses (for example, the rapid rise of gas and oil and food) over which it has little control may allow the quality of its care to suffer in order to live within its budget. On the other hand, alternatives open to an institution may be its use of less expensive medical procedures to hold down costs.

Access

The Act also calls for greater accessibility to services by either high-risk groups such as alcohol and drug abusers, pregnant women over 35 or in their teens, or special groups with traditionally low access to service such as blacks, the elderly, and the poor Spanish-speaking and rural populations. To assist these groups, a number of the HSA plans call for such changes as building clinics in these areas, using ombudspersons to reach out to them, and providing lower cost physician assistants. Regardless of the mechanism used, greater costs will result. Hopefully, savings accrued by the closing of the thousands of acute care beds not needed in the region will be used to pay for these services.

Initial Outcomes of Federal Response to Rising Costs

While it is too early to state clearly that these moves have not worked, early studies raise questions about their ultimate success in curbing costs. Most of the attention has been given to the Certificate-of-Need program. First promulgated by a few pioneering states, it became a national program when built into the health planning act as a required function of HSAs and state health planning agencies. A look at the record thus far indicates that over 90 percent of all proposals reviewed by the HSAs and State Agencies (SAs) are approved.[26] Furthermore, another study shows clearly that while there has been a slowdown in acute care hospital bed growth, there has been no decrease in hospital capital expenditures. This is because the hospitals have shifted their money to purchasing more expensive medical technology.[27] Neither of these trends augur well for the future except that the studies were made before any of the HSA plans were completed. But as noted previously, none of these plans are specific enough to give explicit guidance on what to do with proposals for specialized medical equipment and facilities. The hope is that once such standards are designed and added to the federal minimal guidelines, that there will be an overall decrease in capital expenditures.

With respect to prospective reimbursement, a recent evaluation of the seven experiments indicates that they slowed the rate of increase in hospital costs. The amount of savings, however, is small, compared to the overall cost increases in the health field.[28] In short, it may not make a major contribution in holding down costs.

Regionalization of expensive medical technology has been attempted by some HSAs. Where there already exists an oversupply of such services, it will be difficult to force a hospital or other medical facility to give up an underutilized service. Suggestions to hospitals with vastly underutilized pediatric and obstetric beds to integrate services with other hospitals have met with a chorus of resistance from hospital officials, physicians, and patients accustomed to using those facilities. One can expect similar resistance to HSA plans to reduce the underutilized, costly medical technology of a region. On the other hand, where an undersupply exists, the HSAs and SAs are in a position to make better decisions with respect to the use of new proposed services. However, even if regionalization of medical technology is a success, it will have two potentially negative consequences. First, it will foster the monopoly of these services by medical schools and their teaching hospital affiliates. This may well lead to an emphasis on their use for teaching and research purposes rather than for diagnosis and treatment of illnesses of the general population. Consequently, this could lead to greater inaccessibility for certain populations in the region which traditionally had difficulty being admitted to the prestige hospitals: the poor, the minority patient, and the elderly. Second, it will also lead to increasing the costs of a hospital stay in one of these hospitals. This is understandable in a hospital where the most expensive medical equipment, medical staff, and most difficult-to-treat patients are concentrated. As a corollary of this, a technologic monopoly may lead to the continued deemphasis of physicians practicing in community hospitals. Patients will prefer to be treated at the best medical school and teaching hospitals rather than at the community hospital even though the local institution is more appropriate for their less complicated illnesses.

But, most important of all, the new medical technology has not shown that its use has had any appreciable impact in improving the overall health status of the population. Previously noted studies showed clearly that there was a saving of life for that small portion of the population treated with the latest medical innovations. However, the same study showed that there was a significant increase in most of the diseases being treated by these medical technologies. It is almost like saying that given a vast sum of money I can save 10 lives, but at the same time another 20 persons show up with the same illnesses who cannot be saved. In short, the high cost of medical technology can never win the game if the bottom line requires both a reduction in mortality and morbidity rates. Almost all the medical technologies are used to treat people *after* they become ill. What is being done to help people stay well so they will not require such treatment?

WHAT CAN WE DO?

Collectively, three strategies can make an impact on the reduction of health costs while increasing the health status of the population. These are a medical strategy, a self-help strategy, and a community-based strategy.

Medical Strategy

There is waste and duplication in our medical system. People do become ill and need medical attention. A small portion of these do need to be treated by one of the expensive medical procedures. However, this requires the continued training of biomedically oriented physicians. There has to be a reorientation in medical education so that biomedical training of physicians is not considered the most important educational orientation, but only one of several strands, including family medicine and community medicine. It may be that the medical educators are so wedded to their model of education that they cannot break out of the mold. If that should indeed prove to be the case, then a national health service or a variant may well be needed to overcome the rigidity of medical education.

Second, the expensive medical technology must be rationed and placed where it can best serve the needs of the people, research, and physician education. Recently developed HSA plans appear to be on the right track in their efforts to regionalize these medical technologies. Whether they are best placed in medical schools and teaching hospitals or spread among various hospitals which can become the centers for different specialties has to be discussed and resolved in each region according to its pattern of medical care. In this way, duplication of services will be avoided and the quality of care will be improved because of the full utilization of the available high technology equipment. While the costs may be higher in those institutions with medical specialties, the costs for care in the region will generally be lower. Since the great majority of patients can be treated in community hospitals, it would seem an overall saving of costs will occur in the region.

Although it represents only a start, the guidelines developed by HEW are a good place to begin in the implementation of the regionalization concept:

1. *Bed-population ratio for general hospitals:* Less than four short-term hospital beds per 1000 persons with corrections made for age, seasonal population fluctuations, urban areas, rural areas, and areas with referral hospitals.
2. *Occupancy rate for general hospitals:* An average 80 percent occupancy rate for general, short-term hospitals with corrections for seasonal fluctuations and rural areas.
3. *Obstetrical services:* 2000 deliveries annually in an obstetric unit located in an SMSA (Standard Metropolitan Statistical Area) of 100,000 or more people; average annual occupancy rate of 75 percent with some exceptions for distance.
4. *Pediatric in-patient services; Number of beds:* A minimum of 20 beds in a pediatric unit with some exceptions for distance; the occupancy may vary between 65 percent for small units (20 to 39 beds) and 80 percent for large units (80 or more beds).
5. *Neonatal intensive care units:* Neonatal problem births per 1000 should not exceed four and the unit should have at least 20 beds.
6. *Open heart surgery:* 200 procedures annually, except no new units opened until those existing units perform at least 350 procedures.
7. *Cardiac catherization unit services:* 300 procedures in an adult unit and 150 in a pediatric unit on an annual basis, except no new units opened in a hospital without an open heart surgery unit or until an existing unit performs 500 procedures annually.
8. *Radiation therapy:* A unit to serve a population of 150,000 persons and have at least 450 new cancer cases per year, except no new unit to be started until existing one(s) perform at least 7500 treatments per year.
9. *Computed tomographic scanners:* A unit should perform

2500 procedures per year except no new unit until existing units perform 4500 procedures annually.

10. *End-stage renal dialysis (ESRD):* Should conform to standards and procedures in DHEW regulations governing conditions for coverage of suppliers of ESRD services (20 CFR part 405, Subpart U).

Self-Help Strategy

In recent years, the mass communication media spent considerable time discussing the dangers and symptoms of the three major causes of mortality in this country: heart disease, hypertension, and various forms of cancer. While some may question the nature of the scare tactics used in these health messages, the message has necessarily been received by millions of people. People are more conscious about the suddenness with which their family members, friends, and relatives can die. Noting the poor attention the deceased gave to maintaining their own health prior to their deaths, people may very well have been spurred into examining how they care for their own health and welfare. Whatever the reason, people are more conscious of their health habits and well-being and increasing numbers are doing something about it. Life expectancy among white males increased only about three years between 1900 and 1960. A recent study detailed seven simple exercises, if carried out routinely, would on an average increase a 45-year-old's longevity by about 11 years.[29] Because these seven basic health habits are so simple that anyone can do them without medical guidance, they are worth repeating:

1. Eat three meals a day
2. Eat breakfast every day
3. Engage in moderate exercise two or three times a week such as taking long walks, bicycle riding, swimming, jogging, or gardening
4. Sleep seven to eight hours nightly

5. Refrain from smoking
6. Limit alcohol consumption to one or two drinks at most a day
7. Maintain a moderate weight for your age, height, and bone structure

Of course, those with special addictions or health problems which make it difficult to carry out these seven practices will need special counseling or treatment. As one researcher noted, "increase in life expectancy . . . has been the result primarily of reductions in death rates of early age, not in the lengthening of the normal life span."[30] Implementing these seven health habits speaks exactly to that issue. A 45-year-old man following three or less of these health habits has a life expectancy of 21.6 years whereas a person who practices six or seven of them will have a life expectancy of 33.1 years.[31] None of these seven rules has anything to do with medical technology or high cost of medical care. It is simply a matter of a person caring enough about his or her own well-being.

Community Strategy

A person is not isolated. People live in communities and spend a considerable portion of their lives at work, home, or school and are affected by what happens to them (either subtly or very manifestly) in these places. The noise of horns blowing, machines whirring, the odors of pollutants from chemical plants and waste dumps, and the sour taste of heavily treated water are the more manifest effects on people. More subtly, people are affected by radiation, food preservatives of certain types, dangerous and untreated contaminants in the water, and the routinized tensions of home, work, and educational facilities. While these subtle and manifest elements profoundly influence our physical and mental well-being, they can only be dealt with on a communitywide basis. One individual cannot tell a factory owner to stop polluting the air and the water, a mass transit official that the subways are too noisy, or a teacher or principal that he or she receives too much homework and is served poor quality food in the cafeteria. Collective actions are required to deal with such communitywide problems. While none of the actions has anything to do with medical technology, failure to improve these community problems can only lead to physical and/or mental breakdown requiring medical treatment.

Fortunately for the people in Region II, (New York, New Jersey, Puerto Rico, Virgin Islands) almost all of the HSAs are fully aware of the nature of these problems and have taken the leadership with others to call them to the attention of the public and to try to solve them. An examination of the goals and objectives in some of the Region II HSA plans reveals the following type of positive statements dealing with community problems:

Either fluoridate the local water supply or provide individual mouth rinses to reduce dental defects

Insure that 100 percent of the schoolchildren admitted to school for the first time have been fully immunized

Provide stimulating health education courses that speak to problems dealing with sexual activity, venereal disease, drug and alcohol problems, nutrition, sound dieting techniques, and so forth

Train persons in defensive and safe driving techniques

Train the general public in cardiopulmonary resuscitation techniques

Develop mental health crisis centers in businesses which employ over 400 persons

Educate workers to the potential hazards of their workplace

These represent only a few of the many goals and objectives recommended by these plans. These goals emphasize prevention, health education, and early detection in contrast to the biomedical emphasis in medical education which focuses on diagnosis and treatment.

While no one knows how much it will cost to implement the many changes required in the environment, in our workplaces, and in ourselves, one can anticipate that such changes will be costly. These changes, however, will add a great deal to the overall well-being and health status of the population unlike the emphases on medical technology and treatment procedures. Recommended medical, self-help, and community based strategies should result in a higher cost-benefit ratio and improved health status when compared with data from strictly medical interventions.

In short, there is much more that all of us can do for ourselves. In many instances, people are already doing much more than they did in the past. Credit may not be given to people by persons in authority positions such as physicians, professors, and political leaders. Yet, more and more, the people are becoming the masters of their own well-being.

References

1. Feldstein, M., & Taylor, A. *The rapid rise of hospital costs.* Washington, D.C.: Council on Wage and Price Stability, 1977.
2. Ibid., p. 21.
3. Kissick, W. I. Health policy directions for the 1970's. *New England Journal of Medicine,* 1970, *282*, 1343–54.
4. Feldstein, *Rapid rise,* pp. 31–35.
5. Quote from D. Colman in Fuchs, V. R. *Who shall live?* New York: Basic Books, 1974, p. 28.
6. Ibid., p. 54

7. *Health resources statistics.* Hyattsville, Md.: National Center for Health Statistics, USDHEW, PHS, Health Resources Administration. 1974. Tables 90, 92.
8. Eisenberg, B. S. (Ed.). *Socioeconomic issues of health, '74.* Chicago, American Medical Association, 1974, table 69.
9. Wagner, J., & Zubkoff, M. Medical technology and hospital costs, in M. Zubkoff, I. Raskin, & R. Hanft (Eds.) *Hospital cost containment.* New York: PRODIST, 1978.
10. Selected data from *Health resources statistics.*
11. Leveson, I. Policy issues in evaluation of health technology in R. H. Egdahl, P. M. Gertman (Eds.). *Technology and the quality of health care.* Germantown, Md.: Aspen Systems Inc., 1978, p. 132.
12. *Trends affecting the U.S. health care system.* Cambridge, Mass.: Cambridge Research Institute, 1975, Section III.
13. Feldstein, *Rapid rise*, note 1, Table 10, p. 46 and see text explaining table.
14. Ibid., p. 22
15. Orloff, M. J. Contributions of research in surgical technology to health care, in Egdahl & Gertman, *Technology and the quality of health care,* Tables 6–6 and 6–9.
16. Feldstein, *Rapid rise*, p. 33.
17. Roemer, M. I. *Social medicine.* New York: Springer Pub. Co., 1978, p. 312.
18. Wagner & Zubkoff, *Medical technology,* p. 264.
19. Cambridge Research Institute, *Trends,* pp. 11–12, 13.
20. Fuchs, *Who shall live?*, note 5, p. 64
21. *Computerized tomographic scanning systems.* Cambridge, Mass.: Arthur D. Little, Inc., 1975, Mimeo, unpublished report to Health Resources Administration, DHEW.
22. Orloff, M. J. Contributions of research in surgical technology to health care. In R. H. Egdahl & P. M. Gertman (eds) *Technology and the quality of health care.* Germantown, Md.: Aspen Systems Corp., 1978, Table 6–4, p. 81.
23. Ibid., Table 6–5, pp. 84, 85.
24. Ibid., Banta, H. D., & Sanes, J. R. How the CAT got out of the bag, pp. 185–187.

25. Health Resources Administration. *National guidelines for health planning.* DHEW, Federal Register (NPRM), Washington, D.C.: U.S. Gov't Printing Office, 1977, pp. 485–505.

26. Lewin & Associates. *Evaluation of the efficiency and effectiveness of the section 1122 review process.* Washington, D.C.: September, 1975. (Report to Health Resources Administration, DHEW).

27. Salkever, D., & Bice, T. The impact of certificate of need controls on hospital investment. *Milbank Memorial Fund Quarterly: Health and Society,* 1976, *54,* 185–214.

28. Galbium, T. *Research in health care reimbursement.* DHEW Publication (SSA) 77-11901. Washington, D.C.: U.S. Gov't Printing Office, 1976.

29. Belloc, N. D., & Breslow, L. Relationship of physical health, health status and health practices. *Preventive Medicine,* 1972, (3), 409–421.

30. Fuchs, *Who shall live?* p. 40.

31. Belloc & Breslow, *Physical health status and health practices*, 409–421.

Chapter 13

WORKSHOP SUMMARIES

WORKSHOP 1: THE NEW YORK CITY HEALTH SYSTEMS AGENCY CONSIDERS A BURN UNIT PROPOSAL: A SIMULATION OF AN ACTUAL PROJECT REVIEW

Chairperson: David Smith, J.D.
Executive Committee, HSA
New York, N.Y.

Panelists: Joani George
Deputy Assistant Director for Plan Implementation/Project Review
New York City, HSA

Thomas Miller
Member, HSA Brooklyn District Board
Brooklyn, N.Y.

Eileen Muller
Assistant Director for Plan Implementation/Project Review
New York City HSA

The purpose of this workshop was to illustrate how the HSA obtained a needed burn unit for the New York area. This was achieved without capitulating to several powerful special interests (both consumer and provider) pushing for the approval of a proposal which was less than economically viable.

Workshop panelists (all of whom had been involved in the actual events of the case) reenacted the highly charged, six-hour project review subcommittee meeting. At that meeting the burn-unit application of the Hospital for Plastic and Reconstructive Surgery was examined. The hospital wished to lease space from New York Hospital to operate a 15-unit intensive care burn unit in conjunction with 118 plastic and reconstructive surgery beds. New York Hospital had not yet received approval to construct the eight-story building in which the unit would be housed. Other uses to which this facility would be put had not been specified. The Hospital for Plastic and Reconstructive Surgery planned to help finance the new construction through donations from unnamed contributors in the area. It was argued that the high cost of the burn unit beds would be offset by making the surgical component a "world-renowned" center for plastic surgery in which 95 percent occupancy could be expected.

In the reenactment, panelists Thomas Miller, David Smith, and Joani George closely questioned the applicant (represented by Eileen Muller) as to the financial viability of the project, the need for new as opposed to renovated space, the anticipated occupancy rate, teaching commitments of the institution, and care of the medically indigent. Although the applicant's responses were not found persuasive by the subcommittee, the application was nonetheless approved. Testimony from a wheelchair-bound exfireman, who recounted the severely traumatic experience of having been flown to Texas for burn treatment when nothing was available in the Northeast may have contributed to the decision.

However, the subcommittee was overruled subsequently

by the full project review committee. On the basis of the evidence, the hospital's application was denied. When the matter came before the HSA Executive Committee, a fuller investigation was launched into the matter and the applicant was given further opportunity to defend the application. Ultimately, in spite of a great deal of lobbying by firemen's organizations, the application was turned down by the HSA.

Since the New York regions' need for a burn center was not disputed, the HSA Executive Committee solicited other applicants to fill this gap. Eventually, an application submitted by New York Hospital was approved. A burn unit was installed in renovated facilities there.

Workshop 2: A Medical Center Governing Board Discusses A Family Practice Unit: What Are the Implications for Primary Care? A Simulation

Panelists: Michael Gansl, M.P.H.
Planner, Health and Hospitals Corporation
New York, N.Y.

James Lomax, M.D.
Assistant Director, Family Practice Program
Brookdale Medical Center
Brooklyn, N.Y.

Donald Rubin
President, Consumer Commission on the Accreditation of Health Services, Inc.
New York, N.Y.

Paul Sayegh
Member, Civic Action Group of Cobble Hill, Brooklyn
Brooklyn, N.Y.

Allen D. Spiegel, Ph.D.
Downstate Medical Center, Brooklyn
Brooklyn, N.Y.

In the simulation, Dr. Spiegel played the role of the hospital's board chairman, a banker. Mr. Rubin played an insurance executive and Dr. Lomax played the doctor trying to establish the new program. Mr. Sayegh and Mr. Gansl represented members of the community, a lawyer, and an architect respectively.

Governing board members of a fictitious, prestigious, voluntary nonprofit hospital and medical center discussed the need for a Family Practice Unit (FPU). The idea was presented by the hospital's Director of Ambulatory Care. He is frustrated by his department's inability to deliver primary care given the priorities of the teaching program and subspecialty clinics. This tertiary care facility is located in a racially mixed, "changing" community of middle- to low-income and working poor residents. It is common knowledge that the medical center's staff is resistant to the FPU plan. Staff members believe a family practice plan will reduce revenues, cut into specialty teaching material, and lower hospital prestige. The three "board" members and their chairman argued the points according to their professional priorities. No board member uses the facility for his health care.

Dr. Lomax began his presentation with a criticism of the multi-specialty approach to health care delivery in a community where primary care was needed most. The Emergency Room (ER) became the site for nonemergency care. Holistic care, he argued, was most appropriate for the large majority of community health complaints where the psychosomatic and sociological aspects of illness were as relevant as the organic. An FPU would be cost effective: highly trained specialists would be released from the nonspeciality care they had to deliver in the clinics and ER. And the patient compliance rate is higher when a relationship is established between a family practitioner and families or individuals. Family practice, he said, is its own speciality, despite resistance to it in the Northeastern states.

Dr. Lomax described his plans for unit staffing and training curriculum. In the ensuing debate between Dr. Lomax and the board members issues concerned the cost, the actual impact of the FPU on health status, the nature of the medical center's responsibility to serve the community where it was situated, and the continued ability of the hospital to attract top quality residents into the FPU and specialty programs. Discussion also indicated how varied the definitions of primary care were.

"As someone who has to pay the bills," the insurance executive thought a tertiary care hospital should not be in the business of providing primary and secondary care. A primary care unit should be placed in a community hospital where the reimbursement rate was half that of the medical center. An FPU would only duplicate services and raise costs. The answer was a free-standing facility, offering a prepaid plan—an HMO with a hospital affiliation.

The lawyer, a community resident who agreed to the need for a primary care facility within the community, suggested a satellite center. He, too, was concerned with the indirect costs of a basically soft service in the medical center's hardware atmosphere.

Resistance to the FPU by the medical staff was noted by the architect. He favored the establishment of the unit, but the absence of clear planning criteria disturbed him. Did an FPU meet with the HSA's regionalization plans?

The chairman, a banker, professed that the hospital had a responsibility to the community. However, his comments revealed that he stood with the department chiefs: the specialty clinics could not lose teaching opportunities for their residency programs.

A vote was taken. The Board supported the FPU idea. A committee was appointed to study plans for implementation and to evaluate medical staff support.

WORKSHOP 3: THE NEW YORK CITY HEALTH SYSTEMS AGENCY REVIEWS A PROPOSAL FOR A CYTOGENETIC LABORATORY FOR THE NEW YORK CITY/NEW YORK STATE AMNIOCENTESIS PROJECT: A SIMULATION

Chairperson: Arnold Haber
District Board "A", Queens HSA staff, Data and Special Studies
New York, N.Y.

Panelists: Mary Batten
Chairwoman, Policy and Research Committee of the Prenatal Diagnostic Laboratory of New York City

Rene Jahiel, M.D.
Department of Medicine, New York University Medical Center
New York, N.Y.

Phyllis Klass, M.A., M.S.
Associate Director, Genetic Counselling Program
New York Hospital—Cornell Medical Center
New York, N.Y.

John Steen
Acting Assistant Director, Staten Island HSA Office
New York, N.Y.

Simulation of this 1977 proposal to establish a centralized prenatal cytogenetic diagnostic laboratory followed the normal HSA project review routine. A private, nonprofit agency, the Medical and Health Research Association of NYC, Inc. (MHRA) was the applicant. They asked for permission to renovate a laboratory and purchase appropriate equipment to process amniotic specimens as part of a regionalized program for the prenatal detection of Down's syndrome and neural tube defects in the fetuses of high-risk pregnant women in New York City. This improved, regionalized screening service would accept specimens from all participating regional hospitals offering the surgical service.

Cost containment, based on economies of scale, approximately 4,000 specimens processed a year, and quality control are to be the hallmarks of the service. At least one-half of the total operating expenses of the lab would be covered by third-party payments as projected by the applicant. MHRA predicted that the service could detect and subsequently prevent one-third of the Down's syndrome cases in the city at a savings in social services of $6 to 16 million a year. Six consumers, one 30- to 35-year-old woman from each borough, and a parent of a child with Down's syndrome would join health and science professionals on a unique management advisory committee to determine the direction of the program.

Audience questions following the simulation reflected a concern with the impact of such streamlined screening on the human dimension. For example, would an expansion of screening services increase the number of abortions? Would a noticeable decrease in Down's syndrome in the population actually increase the prejudice against those born with the defect? It was noted that a Committee for Infant Development has been formed to insure maximum support for Down's syndrome children and their families. If the chances for mental growth and development are improved, there may be less need for women to seek termination as the single alternative.

Dr. Jahiel presented an update on the project, scheduled to open in January 1979. He gave four examples of the kind of economic planning that kept the project within its proposed budget: the group purchase by participating hospitals of expensive equipment for the lab, the simple but efficient design of the laboratory itself, and the conversion of existing lab equipment to accommodate new uses.

Workshop 4: Hospital Costs: A Definition of Terms and a Discussion of Issues

Moderator: Edward Gluckmann, M.S.
Executive Vice President
Consumer Commission on the Accreditation of Health Services, Inc.
New York, N.Y.

Panelists: Lawrence Feiner, Ph.D.
Health Care Consultant
New York, N.Y.

Joseph Levi
Director of Financial Planning
Long Island Jewish-Hillside Medical Center
New York, N.Y.

Hospital costs and their effect on the consumer were the theme of this workshop. Dr. Feiner began the panel discussion by comparing the economic trends and practices of the health care industry to those of other industrial enterprises: supply creates demand, what is available will be used. What is remarkable about health care is that its rapid growth has not yet leveled off.

Expanding the industrial analogy, Dr. Feiner said that health services were a product, like plastics. In the health care industry, the number of patients requiring highly technical medical procedures does not support the cost of that technology. Yet, patients get more value out of hospital services than the food consumer receives from a can of Coke. Because competition raises costs, the strong and weak services merge to cut costs. An HMO, for example, is an example of a merger in industrial terms.

Some audience members were disturbed by the comparison of product economics to the health care of people. In answer to a question, Dr. Feiner acknowledged that the health care industry was attractive to investors, that investment capital is attracted to the health care industry and this interest may contribute to high costs. He predicted a leveling off of investments, accompanied by an end to the proliferation of technology.

Mr. Levi wrestled with the problem of hospital charges and actual costs. He cautioned against thinking of cost and charges as interchangeable. In fact, if hospitals charged only the Blue Cross rate, they would not meet their costs. A question came up about indirect costs to the patient such as the training and supervision of interns and residents. Mr. Levi commented that there are specific government rules on cost allocations within a hospital. Hospitals cannot take the blame for operating within these rules. Costs are also raised by the overlapping of so many government regulatory agencies monitoring health care. The health care "mess," he concluded, could be partially solved by restructuring the system of delivery and removing the profit motive. A consumer concurred: the profit motive has blinded administrators to the consumer shift of utilization from inpatient to outpatient services. Costs could be brought down with the provision of more primary care units.

Part IV

THE FUTURE OF MEDICAL TECHNOLOGY

In this concluding conference of the series, an effort was made to look toward the future and to tie all the material from all four conferences into a package designed for follow-up. Therefore, the topics included an emphasis on prevention, reports from two active consumer advocates regarding their practical experiences and the lessons learned, and a proposal that called for public ownership of medical technology. Afternoon workshops also concentrated on this theme by pinpointing the workplace, the aging population, the third-party payers and the concept of regionalization: all future oriented.

Many consumers have contended that it is probably cheaper in the long run to prevent illness than to cure it after the fact. An old maxim reflects this attitude by noting that, "an ounce of prevention is worth more than a pound of cure." Many professionals concur with this approach and several experts during the four conferences attributed the tremendous improvements in health status to improved nutrition, sanitation, and general living conditions as opposed to the benefits occurring from the use of medical technology. Furthermore, the changing pattern of disease in America requires the active participation of the consumer to really have a beneficial impact. People are being afflicted with ailments for which almost no amount of technology will do any good. Only one communicable disease (influenza) is listed among the top 10 killers in America. Other studies have shown that much of the mortality and morbidity is linked to the life-style of the individual. Yet, health care expenditures that are targeted to influence changes in life-style constitute only a small portion of available funds. Most of the funds are expended on existing treatment services where the use of technology is rampant. Have we reached the stage of diminishing returns for our technology dollars? Will the increment in improved health status be so minute as to be unmeasureable? Consumers and providers have to critically examine this view as they make decisions.

However, the reality of health care decision making can not be overlooked. Politics, vested interests, and frank power play a role in considerations about the approval of medical technology. Even though, consumers are mandated by federal law to be at least a majority, and up to 60 percent, of the governing board of an HSA, this does not mean that consumers will vote as a bloc. In fact, one study indicated that the consumers tend to vote the same way as the providers even though they may have more diversity among themselves. In essence, this means that the consumers do not adopt a unified stance in the voting situation. Vested interests may be flagrant among consumers also. Federal law calls for the consumers to represent a diversity of interests including racial, economic, linguistic, geographic, and ethnic groups. Meeting those criteria alone could create adversaries rather than allies among consumer members of the HSA governing boards.

There does seem to be agreement that the future needs some type of organizational effort to inform consumers so they will be better prepared to make decisions about medical technology proposals. This has also been echoed a number of times throughout the four conferences. Providers are able to use existing data sources and are familiar with them from their experiences over the years. Consumers do not have the same access to the data and must rely on their own initiative or the assistance of HSA staff members. Recently, the federal Bureau of Health Planning did issue a notice urging HSAs to assign staff personnel to aid the consumer members. The success of this policy has yet to be demonstrated.

In view of the fragmented health care available in the nation and the failure of efforts to insure adequate care for all, a number of consumer groups envision a national health service or insurance type program in the future. Many who have been active in the field for many years feel that there is no way that powerful health care institutions will yield their domains for the good of the total health care delivery system. No hospital will want to give up its open heart surgery capability. No hospital will want to be the one which sends its patients elsewhere for certain sophisticated laboratory tests. Therefore, it is argued that the only hope will be a governmental health care scheme which forces the powerful institutions to comply through the force of the almighty dollar. This type of inroad is evident in specific governmental programs such as PSROs and surveillance/utilization review activities in Medicaid programs.

Defenders of the current system contend that the pluralistic nature of the health care system ensures that the best care will rise to the top eliminating the inferior services. If any national health scheme does pass through congress, it will incorporate many of the competitive features already extant within the system, according to the organized medical community. Certainly, the future of medical technology is bound up with the fate of these conflicting attitudes and predictions about the health care delivery system as a whole. Consumers must accept the adversary role and press for their desires in much the same style as the providers. Obviously, there are far more consumers so the outcome should be assured. However, providers in this country have a long history of being able to shape the health care system to their own needs regardless of the content of any legislation. Only if health care consumerism matures and coalesces will consumers begin to write a little of their own history.

Milton Terris moved right to the point in the title of his presentation when he stressed health, not illness in talking about prevention in a technologic age. A relationship was established between public health approaches and the use of technology to prevent disease in the future. Using a definition of public health as a foundation, Terris discussed five areas for the future of prevention in a technologic age: sanitation of the environment; control of community disease; education in personal hygiene; personal health services; an adequate standard of living.

Predicting a national department of health, Terris also felt that local health departments will have extraordinary powers. Effects of organizational and legal changes will be reflected in almost complete prevention of disease through contamination of water, food, or milk. Solution of physical and chemical pollution will also be achieved and occupational health problems will be attacked vigorously. Furthermore, city planners will work closely with health departments to assure that human needs are met in housing and environment.

While infectious diseases are already contained to a large degree, Terris forecasted that the second epidemiologic revolution against noninfectious conditions will secure 50 to 75 percent reductions in coronary heart disease, cancer, cerebrovascular disease, obstructive lung diseases, and cirrhosis of the liver. These reductions will take place through shifts in diet, changes in habits, reduced smoking, less alcohol consumption, and the use of new drugs.

Terris expects education in personal hygiene to be stressed in the next century. Funding will be increased greatly, and health education will be conducted on a large scale. In addition, health care providers will learn much more about health education during their student years. Physicians will rely less on drugs and more on giving patients advice, counsel, and education about procedures affecting their health. This will strengthen the physician-patient relationship.

In the realm of personal health services, Terris anticipates that the United States will establish a national health service. Of course, services will be comprehensive and include research, prevention, and care. Yet, there will be increasingly democratic control of health services through citizen boards and councils. Community participation will be encouraged in all phases of the program. Prevention and health promotion will be stressed rather than treatment and diagnosis as is done currently. Interestingly, Terris noted that the national health service will be able to arrange job transfers and changes in living quarters to protect the patient's health.

An adequate standard of living includes an end to unemployment, poverty, and discrimination according to Terris. Much of the violence that abounds in our nation today can be traced to the need for social changes. Should these social changes take place, Terris expects the United States to eclipse completely the remarkable record of the past century in lowering human morbidity and mortality.

Terris concluded with, on a prophetic note: "We stand at the threshold of a great new era. It is our task and our privilege to unlock the door and open it wide to the future."

Speaking from his experience as a consumer activist in Illnois, and particularly in Chicago, Frank Giarrizzo addressed the topic of consumer action in the future. He spoke about the consumer's disappointments in Chicago where political power was the major determinant. In discussing standards for health planning, an article from the *Chicago Sun Times* noted that the Chicago HSA prepared a substandard HSP according to federal government reviewers. Yet, through political power the HSP was approved. Disagreements about hospital bed needs were resolved when a special HSA advisory panel came to the same conclusion as the powerful local hospital council. In addition, virtually all HSA board members and staff are political appointees.

Giarrizzo dealt with these disappointments by suggesting alternative strategies for consumers. He proposed that consumers make their interests felt via the regulatory functions of the state insurance departments and through legislative lobbying. Furthermore, the speaker called on consumers to work to make changes in the federal health planning legislation to shore up the role of the consumer. Also state insurance and finance legislation should be strengthened to provide more protection and participation for and by consumers. Finally, Giarrizzo endorsed the need for an independent consumer network to provide technical and organizational assistance to the consumer sector.

In more of a political vein, Herbert Semmel discussed the reality of health care decision making. Using the example of the CAT scanner, he commented on political decisions, public versus private health perspectives, regulation and decisions, and the need for community organization.

Political decisions should be made through a public process according to Semmel. If this actually occurs, the consumer would have the opportunity to observe the private health perspectives of physicians and hospital administrators. Semmel noted that neither professional is trained to make social decisions and they concentrate on technical reasons for investing in new technology. Relative to the regulation of new technology such as the CAT scanner, Semmel pointed out that the ultimate regulatory power was retained by the state agency where there is much less consumer involvement than in the HSAs.

In conclusion, Semmel spoke about the control of information. He felt that professionals exercised their power through this information control mechanism. He suggested the development of a nationwide network of consumer activist organizations as a possible approach to achieve influence over decisions that literally affect life and death.

John Holloman made a case for public ownership of medical technology in the concluding morning presentation at the fourth conference. He opened by mentioning the objections of some Brooklyn physicians to the care of infants by the New York City Health Department in the early 1900s. Some 30 Brooklyn doctors signed a petition to the Mayor saying that the Health Department was ruining medical practice by keeping babies well and asked that the stations be abolished. Obviously, there was a clash between public interests and private objectives. Expounding on this example, Holloman argued that the public has a moral and practical rationale for owning medical technologic resources. He stated that almost the whole technologic medical care system has been nourished, developed, and supported by public resources and money.

Medical technology in the nation's essentially private enterprise health care system is not provided equally to all. In addition, there appears to be little coordination, and, in fact, the fragmented use of technology may be harming consumers. To resolve this situation, Holloman called for government ownership as the way of removing the profit motive and its devisive goals. Medical technologies would then be distributed with public access in mind and the destructive side effects of competition, such as maldistribution of resources and overdoctoring, would be put to rest.

Finally, Holloman declared that because the public has already paid in large part for the technology, "the least the public can do for itself is to decide how it might best enjoy technological advances and protect itself from technological dangers and abuses."

Afternoon workshops focused on the future theme by discussing how to make the workplace safe, the relationship of the aging population to technology, the future role of third-party payers, and the prospects for regionalization.

A panel presentation reported on efforts to make the workplace safe for workers as well as for the community. There appeared to be no doubt that occupationally related illnesses were a growing problem and that government, in the form of National Institute of Occupational Safety and Health (NIOSH) and Occupational Safety and Health Administration (OSHA), was beginning to take a more active stance in monitoring the workplace environment. Some discussion centered about the relationship of the health care system to occupational illness. Activities for HSAs were also investigated with the suggestion that the HSAs could use the project review process to direct greater attention to the health problems of the workplace.

"Does medical technology hold out any hope for our aging population?" was the question that opened this workshop. After a brief statement of the facts about the aging population, one panelist noted that there was a need for more attention on geriatrics in medical education. Human concern and a caring attitude were also cited as sadly lacking in the selection of health professionals for their roles as healers. One panelist contended that medical care that concentrates on treating organs will not be a major factor in improving the lot of the aging despite the huge medical technologic advances. There has to be more emphasis on improving living standards and the quality of life. This overemphasis on organ-oriented technology is carried over to the awarding of research funds too. Fewer funds are available for human and social services needed by the aged. These societal decisions could be altered if the aged were more extensively organized and their political power brought to bear on those who allocate resources.

In the panel discussion on the role of third-party payers and their impact on technology, Eugene Sibery said, "Health care goals and needs cannot keep up with advances in diagnosis and treatment. New procedures—expensive and needlessly applied—combined with the proliferation of specialized manpower have contributed to uncontrollable costs." Loopholes in the Certificate-of-Need process and existing third-party reimbursement procedures were cited as actually having stimulated technologic expansion. The typical third-party policy of retrospectively reimbursing a hospital's operating costs was called "the blank check theory" by one panelist who accused the insurance industry of uncritically underwriting health care expansion at the expense of the consumer. Adequate record keeping, second opinions, hold harmless clauses, and a watchdog role on standards for third-party payers were also discussed as solutions for misutilization and high costs in health care.

Regionalization concepts, myths and reality was the topic for another workshop. Opening the session, the question was posed, "Can regionalization be implemented in our present system or is total reform necessary?" In response, one panelist suggested that the Certificate-of-Need program was a key strategy in realizing regionalization within the current system. Misconceptions about regionalization and a lack of uniform definitions of basic concepts such as primary, secondary, and tertiary care were clarified. The British health care approach was explained and consumers in the audience asked panelists about the prospects for an American national health service. Power struggles within the HSAs and the provider dominance of planning activities were also discussed. While the discussion was intense, no resolution to regionalization was forthcoming except for the prediction that a regionalized system would eventually become a reality.

Chapter 14

HEALTH, NOT ILLNESS: PREVENTION IN A TECHNOLOGIC AGE

Milton Terris

It is safe to say that in the next century, unless we succeed in destroying ourselves, changes in our way of life will be even greater, perhaps exponentially greater, than in the preceding century. A major reason is the scientific and technological revolution; we stand today only on its threshold. Another reason is the evolution of public health, which refuses to stand still. Finally, the whole of society is changing, and this change will profoundly affect health care in myriad ways.

Dr. Stephen Smith,[1] the founder and first President of the American Public Health Association, declared at its first annual meeting in 1873 that

> the science which we cultivate, and which this Association is organized to promote, discarding the traditions of the past and the teachings of false philosophies, interprets the laws that have been set for the guidance and control of man's earthly existence by the exact demonstrations of a true physiology. This science

[1]Reprinted from Milton Terris, "Public Health in the United States: The next 100 years," *Public Health Reports, 93 (6): 602–606, 1978. Used with permission.*

> of life reveals to us the stupendous fact that man is born to health and longevity, that disease is abnormal, and death, except from old age, is accidental, and that both are preventable by human agencies.

This was a statement of faith and a prediction: faith in the liberating power of science and a prediction of its enormous potential for preventing disease and death. Effective use of that potential by health workers during the past 100 years is unquestionably one of the great and inspiring chapters in the history of mankind.

Perhaps the best way to approach these prospects is in terms of C. E. A. Winslow's[2] definition of public health which, though formulated more than half a century ago, remains to this day the most thoughtful and inclusive:

> Public health is the science and the art of preventing disease, prolonging life, and promoting physical health and efficiency through organized community efforts for the sanitation of the environment, the control of community infections, the education of the individual in principles of personal hygiene, the organization of medical and nursing service for the early diagnosis and preventive treatment of disease, and the development of the social machinery which will ensure to every individual in the community a standard of living adequate for the maintenance of health.

Winslow's definition of public health is unusual on several counts: First, it emphasizes the promotion of health as well as the prevention of disease. Second, it is concerned with the preventive values of early diagnosis and treatment. Third, it recognizes the need to develop "the social machinery which will ensure to every individual in the community a standard of living adequate for the maintenance of health." Five areas listed in his definition provide a comprehensive and logical framework for discussion of the future of prevention in a technologic age.

Sanitation of the Environment

During the next 100 years, sanitation of the environment will cease to be a stepchild and become, as it was until recent years, a major activity of health departments. Health departments will be radically reorganized. There will be a Department of Health at the federal level, responsible for basic national policies and standards for all public health programs, including those concerned with environmental health. Health departments at the state and local levels will be responsible for carrying out national policies and maintaining national standards; their jurisdiction will include all environmental health programs, such as air and water pollution, sewage disposal, milk and food sanitation, radiation, occupational disease and injuries, automotive and other accidents, and drugs, food additives, and other chemicals that adversely affect the environment.

Local health departments will have extraordinary powers. No residential, industrial, or institutional construction will be permitted without prior determination by the health department that it meets approved health and safety standards. These standards will be concerned not only with preventing disease and injury but also with positive health, for example, with temperature, noise, and other factors in comfort, efficiency, and well-being.

State and local health departments will have similar powers of approval for the construction of new roads and the improvement of old ones. Indeed, one of their tasks will be to study existing roads to determine the presence of hazards; the health departments will also have the authority to order their abatement. Hazards resulting from errors in the construction of automobiles, trucks, buses, tractors and other farm machinery, airplanes, and other vehicles will be dealt with by the federal Department of Health in cooperation with state health departments.

Occupational health services, which are only now beginning to come into their own in the United States, will be an important aspect of environmental control by local, state, and federal health departments. Again, these departments will have the power not only to study and inspect, but also to order the removal of hazards. To provide the scientific basis for these programs, there will be a considerable expansion of research institutes concerned with different aspects of environmental health. These institutes will be constructed by federal and state health departments in various parts of the country rather than being concentrated in one or two places.

What will be the effects of these organizational and legal changes? Coupled with substantial increases in funds for environmental health, they may be expected to result in almost complete prevention of contamination of water, milk, and food with disease-producing microorganisms. Technical problems of physical and chemical pollution of air and water will most certainly be solved, as will those of solid waste disposal. Protection against radiation and nuclear energy will be made almost foolproof.

There will be a sharp drop in occupational injuries, and ways will be found to protect workers against known agents of occupational disease. It is the unknown agents that will continue to create problems, as well as the host of new chemicals that will be created for use in industry, medicine, food, clothing, and housing. Although every effort will be made to devise rapid and effective tests of these chemicals for possible harmful effects, that may not always be possible because of the long "incubation period" before some of the effects appear.

Accidents will be greatly reduced by thorough and continuing attention to the agent, host, and environmental factors involved. One hundred years from now, people will be shocked to find that in 1978 accidents were the fourth leading cause of death in the United States.

City planners will work closely with their health department colleagues to assure that cities and their rural surroundings are planned for maximum human comfort, efficiency, and well-being. In 100 years, during which our society will have become fully geared to planning for human needs, slums will have disappeared. Only older buildings of historical interest will have been kept; all others will have been constructed to meet health department specifications with regard to light, ventilation, temperature, noise, and size of rooms. In addition, the rational use of space for dwellings, recreational green belts, and industrial areas will have become a major focus of attention for both city planners and health workers.

Control of Community Diseases

Writing in 1923, long before the development of epidemiologic research in the noninfectious diseases, Winslow limited the control of disease to community infections. The past 100 years have seen the virtual completion of this first epidemiologic revolution: the conquest of the infectious diseases. Even though the control of a number of these diseases, such as influenza, the common cold, and the venereal diseases, remains elusive, there is every reason to believe that improved scientific tools and control methods will be developed to cope with them.

Control of noninfectious diseases, the second epidemiologic revolution, has already begun. Whether this revolution will also be completed virtually within 100 years is difficult to say. On the other hand, there is no doubt that major declines in the most significant noninfectious diseases will be achieved. From 50 to 75 percent of the morbidity and mortality from such leading causes of death as coronary heart disease, cancer, cerebrovascular disease, chronic obstructive lung disease, and cirrhosis of the liver will be prevented.

The reduction in coronary heart disease will be achieved by a shift in the American diet from saturated to unsaturated fats, by effective programs for the detection and treatment of hypertension, and by measures to lessen the prevalence and amount of cigarette smoking. Much cancer will be prevented by environmental control of exposure to specific carcinogens in the workplace and the general environment and by a variety of economic, regulatory, and educational measures to discourage cigarette and alcohol use. A large portion of cerebrovascular disease will be prevented by massive programs for the detection and continued treatment of hypertension. Chronic obstructive lung disease will decrease in direct proportion to the decline in cigarette smoking.

Cirrhosis of the liver will likewise decrease in direct proportion to the decline in alcohol consumption. There is no reason to believe that we cannot repeat the British experience. Through a policy of increasing taxation, the price of alcohol rose in the United Kingdom by 4½ times from 1918 to 1936.[3] In this period, the consumption of alcohol declined by two-thirds in England and three-fourths in Scotland. By 1936, the death rate for cirrhosis of the liver was down to 3 per 100,000 as compared with 10 per 100,00 in 1914—a 70 percent decrease. And this lowered mortality rate has been maintained ever since. The death rate in the United States for cirrhosis of the liver now stands at 15 per 100,000, slightly higher than it was in 1914; a reduction equivalent to that of the United Kingdom would bring it down to less than 5 deaths per 100,000.

High mortality diseases, such as diabetes and cancers of certain sites, remain, and current knowledge is inadequate for either prevention or treatment. There are also others that cause a great deal of disability but do not kill, such as arthritis and mental disorders, for which, again, our knowledge is incomplete. However, it is difficult to believe that this situation will remain static. Recent findings that lithium is a preventive agent in manic depressive disease mark an important breakthrough. Sooner or later other breakthroughs will occur as a result of the rapidly increasing tempo of scientific research.

Education in Personal Hygiene

During the latter decades of the past century, health education came to be deemphasized, disparaged, and almost completely disregarded. In large measure this situation resulted from the efficacy of technical measures such as immunization and environmental control in the prevention of infectious diseases.

Prevention of the noninfectious diseases requires a high degree of understanding and cooperation from the individual. Therefore, in this era of the second epidemiologic revolution, health education will occupy a central rather than a peripheral position in health practice. Health education will prove essential also because without an informed public, it will be impossible to institute the necessary measures to protect individuals from health hazards in their physical and social environments.

Health education in the next 100 years will be well financed and conducted on a large scale. It will also be highly sophisticated, using all the techniques developed by our modern media. But it will not stop there. For example, health education will no longer be a hit or miss program in the schools, but will become an important aspect of the curriculum, taught by sufficient numbers of well-trained, full-time personnel.

Even more important, health education will assume its rightful place in the curriculum of schools of the health professions. All health workers—physicians, dentists, nurses, social workers, nutritionists, psychologists, and so forth—regardless of their position in the health care system, will be expected to spend a certain amount of their working time in health education. This time will be used in giving lectures or talks to community organizations, conducting classes for parents or for groups with specific chronic diseases, or preparing written materials. In addition, all health workers engaged in the direct care of patients will be expected to discuss the patients' health problems with them, give them advice and counsel, and teach them how to promote health and prevent disease.

In so doing, health workers will be heeding the conclusions of an important, but curiously disregarded, study that appeared many years ago.[4] Comparing medical groups that had different levels of hospital training after graduation, the Public Health Serivce found a positive correlation between length of hospital training and diagnostic thoroughness: the groups with the most hospital training performed more general, more rectal, and more x-ray examinations. Far more interesting was the finding that the groups with the least hospital training had a greater tendency to prescribe sedatives or stimulants, topical applications, vitamins, hormones, and cathartics. On the other hand, the groups with the most hospital training were more likely to recommend bed rest or exercise or to give advice relating to diet.

Implications are clear enough. More highly trained physicians rely less on drugs and more on giving patients advice, counsel, and education about procedures affecting health. Improvement in the quality of health care will mean a weakening of physicians' overdependence on drugs (their drug culture, so to speak) and a strengthening of the patient–physician relationship through discussion, advice, and health education. Undoubtedly, the next 100 years will see great strides in this direction.

Personal Health Services

After a distressing period of experimentation with private and governmental health insurance—in which bureaucracy will increase as a result of vain attempts to contain costs, and inequitites in health service will continue—the United States will establish a National Health Service.

This National Health Service will have three major components: research, disease prevention, and personal health services (health care). A research component will be comprised of the National Institutes of Health, including new institutes that will have been set up in different parts of the country. Disease prevention will include all programs for the prevention and control of infectious and noninfectious diseases and trauma. In accordance with the policy of recognizing the primacy of prevention, this component will receive a great deal of budgetary and organizational emphasis.

The health care component will serve the entire population, except for a small proportion of people who prefer to use private physicians. Even this small proportion will have dwindled to practically zero by the end of the 100-year period.

Services will be comprehensive and will include mental, dental, and long-term care. There will be no payments by patients for any of the services. These will be provided in community health centers and hospitals staffed by salaried physicians and other salaried health workers. Furthermore, the National Health Service will make possible the establishment of a national network of medical institutions. This dream of regionalization so remarkably well conceived by Dr. Joseph W. Mountin and his colleagues in the 1940s,[5,6] will now be realized. In accordance with patients' needs, they will be referred from small hospitals to larger and more specialized institutions, and eventually if necessary to university medical centers. Health personnel will move in this direction for postgraduate education at the complete expense of the National Health Service. In the other direction, personnel from the university medical centers and the more specialized institutions will visit the smaller hospitals to provide consultation and education.

State and local health departments will be part of the National Health Service, responsible to it in the area of overall policy and standards, but responsible to their respective state and local governments for the effectiveness of the services provided. Like the National Health Service, the state health departments will maintain the three basic components of research, disease prevention, and health care; local health departments will usually be concerned only with disease prevention and health care.

Bureaucratic morasses resulting from a plethora of specialized and fragmentary health programs and the enormous paper work involved in fee-for-service payment for health services will disappear. The federal health establishment will actually shrink after the National Health Service is established, since it will be concerned primarily with the development of policy; implementation will occur primarily at the local level and secondarily at the state level for regional coordination.

There will be increasingly democratic control of health services. All health departments and institutions will be responsible to boards or councils representing all sections of the population. This situation will be in sharp contrast to the present one, in which relatively small sections of the population dominate the boards of hospitals, health departments, and voluntary health agencies.

Perhaps even more important, the public will be drawn into the work of health departments on a scale far greater than in the past. This involvement will be common particularly in programs for the prevention of infectious and noninfectious diseases and trauma, but will also be common in health care. Community organizations and individual volunteers will play an important role in providing assistance to health personnel in health education, immunization campaigns, and environmental health, occupational health and safety, mass screening, and first aid. Such participation will not only strengthen health programs, but will give the public a much greater understanding of the needs and problems of the health services.

Medical services will also change. It is unwarranted to describe current medical services as "health care"; what we now provide is, for the most part, diagnosis and treatment. With the exception of pediatrics and obstetrics, little emphasis is put on the promotion of health and the prevention of disease. Yet Winslow, in his definition, not only defines "promoting physical health and efficiency" as a basic objective, but includes medical care in a specific conceptual framework, namely "the organization of medical and nursing service for the early diagnosis and preventive treatment of disease."

The National Health Service will be oriented toward health promotion as well as toward the early diagnosis and preventive treatment of disease. In the health promotion area, the physicians, nurses, and other health personnel will be particularly concerned with the growth and development of children. They will want to assure that both children and adults have the adequate diets, sufficient sleep, rest and recreation, and optimal exercise that will not only help prevent illness but will result in positive health, that is, vigor, energy, and vitality.

Early diagnosis and preventive treatment will be extended through automated multiphasic screening methods to the entire population. They will be extended beyond disease detection to include the detection of risk factors such as elevated serum cholesterol. Follow-up will be intensive in order to assure that the needed treatment is instituted.

Supervision to maintain adequate health of pregnant women, infants, children, workers in hazardous occupations, and people with chronic diseases will become an accepted part of the health services. Every attempt will be made, including home visits when necessary, to have people remain under appropriate supervision and care. Furthermore, the health services will not only have the authority to prescribe the environmental changes needed to protect the patient's health, including job transfers and changes in living quarters, but will also have the authority to get the prescription filled by the responsible agency.

An Adequate Standard of Living

Winslow saw clearly the close relationship between poverty and disease.[7] Therefore, it is not surprising that he included in his definition "the development of the social machinery which will ensure to every individual in the community a standard of living adequate for the maintenance of health."

Poverty and its too-constant partner, discrimination, are responsible for a great deal of unnecessary disease. They are also at the root of much of the violence that threatens all classes of the population in our cities. Just as cholera in the 19th century moved out of the hovels of the poor to reach into the homes of the well-to-do, so violence today moves out of the slums and the ghettos to make entire cities unsafe.

Therefore, from a public health viewpoint, it will become necessary for society to bring an end to unemployment, poverty, and discrimination, and to assure satisfactory pensions for the retired instead of the current crazy quilt of inadequate programs. There can be no doubt that these changes will be accomplished in the next 100 years. As with all significant social changes, we must be concerned that they be consummated with as little travail as is humanly possible.

Once these changes occur, the way will be open for an unprecendented advance in the health of the public. Together with effective control of environmental hazards, large-scale programs against noninfectious diseases and trauma, intensive and extensive use of health education, rational organization of medical services and the transformation of these services into health care, and future discoveries that we may confidently expect as a result of the burgeoning scientific and technologic revolution, these economic and social changes will make it possible in the next 100 years for the United States to eclipse completely its remarkable record of the past century in lowering human morbidity and mortality.

We stand at the threshold of a great new era. It is our task and our privilege to unlock to door and open it wide to the future.

References

1. Smith, S. Public health reports and papers presented at the meetings of the American Public Health Association in the year 1873. New York: Hurd and Houghton, Riverside Press, 1874.
2. Winslow, C. E. A. *The evolution and significance of the modern public health campaign.* New Haven, Conn.: Yale University Press, 1923.
3. Terris, M. Epidemiology of cirrhosis of the liver: National mortality data. *American Journal of Public Health,* 1967, *57,* 2076–2088.

4. Ciocco, A., Hunt, G. H., & Altman, I.: Statistics on clinical services to new patients in medical groups. *Public Health Reports,* 1950, *65,* 99–115.

5. Mountin, J. W., Pennel, E. H., & Hoge, V. M. *Health service areas, requirements for general hospitals and health centers.* Public Health Bulletin No. 292. Washington, D.C.: U.S. Public Health Service, 1945.

6. Mountin, J. W. & Greve, C. H. *Public health areas and hospital facilities, A plan for coordination.* Washington, D.C.: Public Health Service Publication No. 42. 1950.

7. Winslow, C. E. A. Poverty and disease. *American Journal of Public Health,* 1948, *38,* 173–184.

Chapter 15

CONSUMER ACTION FOR HEALTH IN THE FUTURE: AN ILLINOIS PERSPECTIVE

Frank C. Giarrizzo

Passage by Congress in 1974 of Public Law 93–641, the National Health Planning and Resources Development Act, raised high hopes among consumer health activists that finally our nation's medical care problems might be brought under control. One of the major goals of the Act was the development of a comprehensive and effective planning structure, with consumers mandated to play a leading role in developing plans and implementing programs. Because of its great promise to help improve the nation's health status, the new legislation was supported enthusiastically by consumer health activists everywhere.

Consumer Disappointments

Consumer activists in Illinois have experienced some disappointments with health planning. I will describe a few of the strategies we have developed to compensate for many of the deficiencies in the law. Then, I will conclude with few of my own recommendations for consumer health action in the future that have evolved from these experiences.

As we approach the end of the third full year of health planning under P.L. 93–641, the aims of many consumers have been largely unfulfilled. There is a great deal of skepticism in some consumer quarters regarding the prospects of health planning to succeed. In Illinois, and particularly in the city of Chicago, consumer health activitists have become increasingly concerned and disillusioned. They are seeking alternative solutions to health planning problems. I am convinced that many of these problems are not unique to our community. We must begin to develop new strategies for future action if suitable solutions are to be found.

Standards for Planning

Consider just a few of the concerns, particularly the level of performance of health planners and their responsiveness to consumer interests. We are told that the main function of health planners is the development of plans and the implementation of programs so that each health planning area's needs and priorities may be identified, and appropriate types of services can be established, expanded, or limited. Obviously, the level of performance can be expected to vary somewhat from one area to another. One might also expect, however, that some minimal, uniform standards would be used consistently in determining whether or not an agency is achieving the objectives of the law.

Conclusions of a panel of federal government experts on the product of the Chicago health system agency's planning efforts supply an indication. Standards being used have less to do with the ability of the agency to do the planning job than with political considerations, a problem not unique to our part of the country. In their Sunday, November 5, 1978 issue, the *Chicago Sun Times* disclosed how politics govern planning decisions when it printed the contents of an HEW staff report on its evaluation of the Chicago HSA's Health System Plan. This newspaper article stated:

> The (Chicago HSA) plan ignored virtually every component of the health care delivery system except facilities operated by the Chicago Board of Health—like the HSA, a politically dominated agency answerable to City Hall. The plan made no mention of either private doctors' offices, or varied programs offered by the Cook County Health and Hospitals Governing Commission, which has been politically independent of organization Democrats since 1969.

It might be noted that the Governing Commission operates Cook County Hospital, Chicago's only public hospital and the largest provider of medical services to the sick poor. The *Sun Times* article went on to report, "The plan ignored factors affecting exposure to injury and disease of employees in the workplace. The agency made only a 'limited' attempt to explore how Chicagoans use the health system, habits whose analysis is seen by federal health planners as the key to the careful mapping of change." In conclusion, the six page internal HEW report commented that the Chicago HSA had spent $1.5 million in federal funds to draw up a health plan for the city that was found to be unacceptable.

Under the Freedom of Information Act, the report of the federal review panel was voluntarily released by HEW to the *Sun Times* after a federal investigation was begun into the reasons behind HEW's approval of permanent designation status for the Chicago HSA as a planning agency. The Chicago HSA contract was awarded by HEW despite the unanimous opinion of its own panel of experts that the Agency's Health System Plan should be rejected. In addition, this action took place despite vigorous objections of Chicago consumer health activists who had previously been critical at every level of the health planning review process.

Disagreement on Bed Needs

Yet, the Chicago HSA is not alone in having problems developing health plans and in determining the city's health needs and priorities. In regard to bed need determination, local, state, and even federal health planners seem to be having trouble agreeing on the appropriate level of waste to be allowed. For example, according to federal government bed-need computations, Chicago has as many as 8,155 excess hospital beds out of a total of 20,057 beds in place. The state of Illinois Certificate-of-Need agency estimates 5,760 unneeded beds. Just recently, a special Chicago HSA advisory panel identified only 1,313 beds as being unnecessary. Not surprisingly, the politically influential local hospital council had earlier concluded there were between 1,400 and 1,700 unneeded beds, a figure remarkably close to the city administration's estimate.

Participation by Consumers and Politics

Consider as a further example of unfulfilled aims of consumer health activists, the failure to promote more effective consumer participation in health planning decisions. Consumer aims of P.L. 93–641 seem to be clear. This Act emphasizes public notice and open hearings, local accountability and consumer involvement. P.L. 93–641 states that consumers should be "broadly representative of the social, economic, linguistic and racial population of the health service area." Consumer involvement is considered "essential to the effective performance of an agency's function." Further, consumer majorities are mandated on decision-making bodies at all levels of health planning.

Today, some health system areas seem to be no closer to realizing the goal of effective consumer participation in health planning than when the legislation was first enacted into law.

For example, the Los Angeles HSA recently had its contract terminated because a Government Accounting Office audit was sharply critical of political favoritism than shaped the hiring policy of the agency. This agency was also cited for its lack of accountability to consumer interests. In rural Champaign County, Illinois, the local HSA is now on a one-year probationary status because of its lack of accountability to consumer interests. It was only after a prolonged two-year battle led by consumer activists, that legitimate consumer representatives were able to replace provider sponsored members on the local board.

In Chicago, virtually all HSA board members and staff are political appointees. According to the previously mentioned *Sun Times* report, the HSA even went so far as to return $100,000 to the federal government in order to avoid setting up subarea advisory councils in the city's neighborhoods. Sources inside the HSA were quoted as saying "the program was scrapped when city hall officials complained that public participation would mean effective consumer control of the agency." An HEW insider reportedly stated the highest ranking HEW official in Washington had ordered full designation after city hall pressure was brought to bear in Washington.

Obviously these are some of the worst cases. Many HSAs are admittedly having greater success doing their job. Yet, many of the consumer board members I have talked with around the country consider their efforts as merely "tinkering" with the system. Some even suspect they are just being "used" by providers and government bureaucrats.

Alternative Strategy— Insurance Departments

While there is disillusionment with the slow progress of health planning, particularly in Illinois, some significant headway has fortunately been made in other health regulatory areas. The largest gains have been made in Illinois Insurance Department hearings reviewing the operations of Blue Cross/Blue Shield of Chicago, the state's largest health care insurer. Illinois consumer activists have been able to address health issues through these actions that are completely out of the jursidiction of health planning agencies.

Main issues in the "Blues" hearings have focused on two broad areas. The first involves the internal financial needs of the "Blues"; specifically, the actuarial and mathematical soundness of their filed rates, the reasonableness of projected surpluses and the costs incurred in the solicitation of business. The second, and most interesting broad issue, concerns the adequacy of the "Blues" efforts in the promotion or preservation of their subscribers' mental and physical health.

A result of consumer intervention in the hearings was a complete denial of rate increase requests and a long series of orders to the "Blues" to institute programs and policies that would benefit their subscribers. The "Blues" have been ordered to renegotiate their 28-year-old contracts with Illinois hospitals. New contracts must include provisions requiring them to provide a mechanism that would prospectively assess the reasonableness of a hospital's financial requirements and its rate structure. Using a new consumer sponsored law, the insurance director would be able to monitor the "Blues" activities in this area. In addition, the director would be able to contain rates of reimbursement not only to hospitals but also to other participating health care providers.

A total of 16 orders have been imposed on the "Blues" specifying programs that would expand subscriber rights; develop stringent standards for utilization review; require plans to be drawn up to reduce excess hospital capacity; expand extended care and coordinated home care services, preadmission testing, outpatient surgery, second opinions on surgery, provider education services; and would help implement state mandated generic drug programs. Nonhospital providers were also affected as they were ordered to negotiate new contracts which must include hold-harmless agreements that protect subscribers from being charged for hospital and physician services the "Blues" refused to pay.

In short, because of the insurance department legal interventions, consumers have made inroads in areas that health planners do not get into in their wildest dreams. Here, the consumer strategy has been relatively simple. The Chicago "Blues" were selected as a target because they account for almost 50 percent of the revenue of 300 hospitals in the state, 20 percent of which is federal Medicare money. "Blues" are chartered under their own unique not-for-profit insurance law, which made it possible for consumers to oppose them in a one-on-one confrontation in the hearings. However, the economic leverage this one insurer holds over medical providers in the state was the most significant factor influencing consumers in their decision to mount a legal offensive in the hearings.

Legislation Alternative

A significant fall-out of the insurance hearings has been the enactment of a new state law establishing a prospective rate review authority in Illinois. Previously, the state hospital association opposed an earlier version dating back to 1970 that would have given the state the power to approve hospital budgets each year. When it became apparent that the insurance director was going to force Blue Cross to review budgets if another state agency did not, the hospital association sat down with health insurers and drafted their own version. Some consumers opposed the final legislation, because it guaranteed equitable treatment for hospitals but did not provide sufficient cost containment guarantees for the public. Consumer activists were able to rewrite about 20 percent of the bill's language so as to strengthen it somewhat.

Hopefully, the experiences of consumers in Illinois in dealing with health regulatory agencies should convince consumer activists elsewhere with similar problems that victories can be won despite the odds. Strategies and actions employed in Illinois can be implemented in every state in the union.

Improve P.L. 93–641

But there are other things that must be done too. Specifically, those concerned with consumer involvement in health planning must work to amend and strengthen P. L. 93–641. Further, neither providers, nor public entities with documented histories of abuses in inplementing consumer participatory programs must be allowed to control health planning agencies. We must see to it that there are truly independent HSAs, with improved board election procedures in every area. Consumer members should be provided with their own staff and receive educational support services so that HSA can begin to serve as a forum for broader dialog with each other. We must reduce the power of the provider groups so that the present imbalance between provider and consumer interests is corrected. We must see to it that the planning law is extended far beyond the current one-year period that American Medical Association lobbyists have forced upon us through their influence in Congress.

Strengthen Insurance and Finance Laws

Next, state, insurance and health finance laws must be amended and strengthened. Loopholes that allow medical care insurers to pass through unreasonable costs unchallenged to subscribers must also be closed. We must begin a campaign of payment containment, not just cost containment. All regulatory agencies should be forced to deny rate increases to third-party payers if they fail to make a vigorous, good-faith effort to contain rates of reimbursement to providers. Consumers should see to it that regulatory agencies promote cost-effective alternative forms of care. All of the health finance mechanisms and insurance regulatory agencies in the nation must then be brought under one umbrella, just as has been done with the health planning agencies.

Independent Consumer Health Network

Finally, a powerful and independent consumer health network must be built that would advocate a national health plan to provide medical care to everyone, without exception. A key ingredient of the plan must be a program that would attempt to make us all less reliant on the medical care industry for our health. There is no substitute for a population that is knowledgeable in the fact that prevention, health maintenance, and community-based primary care are the real secrets to better health.

Chapter 16

THE REALITY OF HEALTH CARE DECISION MAKING

Herbert Semmel

How are decisions on medical technology made? Health care decision making can be illustrated by the case of the CAT scanner.

POLITICAL DECISIONS

Already, the American people are obligated to pay over two billion dollars for CAT scanners. Before the "demand" is satisfied, the total will reach three to four billion. Initial outlays are made by hospitals and physicians, but the ultimate payment comes from the public through health insurance premiums and taxes which pay the charges imposed for use of the scanners. Decisions to spend billions on CAT scanners evolved from literally hundreds of private decisions made by hospitals and physicians. These decisions were supplemented by limited participation of state health planning agencies in states having Certificate-of-Need or 1122 programs.

Decisions as to whether to spend money on CAT scanners

are political as they involve the allocation of limited resources. Recent proposals of the Carter administration to slash health expenditures as well as other human services is a reminder of how real these limitations are, even with 9 percent of our gross national product going for health care. Monies spent on scanners ultimately compete with funding on cancer research, the availability of home health services, the development of preventive health services, rural health initiatives and primary care clinics, and, in the broadest sense, with expenditures to improve health by reducing environmental pollution.

Political decisions should be made through a public process. Why was the allocation of billions for CAT scanners made privately? At the time the CAT scanner boom started in the early to middle 1970s, there was little in the way of a legal structure which imposed public planning or control. Certificate-of-Need laws were either nonexistent or weak, doctors' offices were not covered in any case, and planning agencies were provider dominated. Despite changes introduced by the National Health Planning and Resources Development Act of 1974, the situation remains basically the same today.

Public Versus Private Health Perspective

It is interesting to inquire as to what the doctors and hospitals administrators knew about CAT scanners when the decisions to invest billions were made. They knew that, in certain special cases, remarkable diagnostic results could be achieved. It was not known to what extent these diagnostic improvements affect health outcomes. For example, identification by a CAT scanner of an otherwise undetectable brain tumor does not effect outcome if the tumor cannot be treated. Nor do physicians consider alternative health uses of the funds which are to be used to purchase scanners. They are not trained to do so, nor does the practice of medicine generally develop a public health perspective in the physician. A physician has a private health perspective, which focuses on crisis intervention and a relatively small group of individual patients for whom the physician feels personally responsible. In these circumstances, the decision to utilize a new instrument of technology is an easy one, if a payment mechanism is available. When faced with a sick human being for whom no diagnosis or treatment seems effective, utilization of a new technique for that individual seems to make sense, regardless of whether the outcome will be affected in only 1 case in 50, 500, or 5000. That patient is a human whose life might be saved. Furthermore, the satisfaction to the physician of saving that patient is great. If the patient is lost, any self-doubts and any malpractice claims are dispelled by having tried "everything."

Hospital administrators are hardly in a better position to make social decisions. Their responsibility is to their institutions. Their decisions have little or no regard for general health needs of the public, particularly those needs unrelated to hospital care. Careers of hospital administrators, particularly in the dominant voluntary sector, are best advanced by expansion of building and "modernization." A new wing is a permanent tribute to the skill of the administrator.

Since doctors admit patients, hospitals cater to doctors. If doctors want a scanner, the hospital will provide one. Otherwise, a "competing" hospital will, or some doctors will buy one of their own. Once installed, the scanner is used sufficiently to pay for itself, no matter how many are already in operation in the area.

Regulation and Decisions

As the demand for public control of scientific policy decision making increases, a new phenomenon has arisen, that of regulation by experts. Rather than true public accountability and control, a process develops in which lip service in institutional form is given to a public process. In reality, the staff of the new regulatory agencies exercise the the actual power.

This trend is becoming most evident in the health planning

field. A great deal of publicity is given the HSAs, and to their "broadly representative" consumer majorities. But the reality is that the greater power is retained by the State Health Planning and Development Agencies, state agencies staffed by professional planners with no citizen involvement. Currently, the greatest power possessed by planning agencies is the Certificate-of-Need and this power lies in the state agency. In effect, institutions need a license to make capital expenditures. Properly utilized, the power to grant or deny a Certificate-of-Need can have substantial impact on allocation of resources. HSAs play only an advisory role in the certificate of need process. HSAs do adopt the Health Systems Plan (HSP). There is no legal requirement that the state agency adhere to the HSP in Certificate-of-Need decisions. At the HSA level, traditional provider dominance still prevails in many areas. In others, it has often been replaced by the domination of the professional planners who are often well meaning; they believe they have the knowledge and the ability to make the best judgments. Members of the public, consumer and providers alike, serving on the boards and committees are viewed by the planners as chess pieces to be moved about to provide support for the planners' decisions. Planners have a virtual monopoly on information and training, particularly vis-à-vis consumers. And consumers are acting as volunteers, with limited time to devote.

In the planning process, the role which planners should play is to present to the public representatives (in understandable form) the issues, alternatives, and consequences of the decisions that are to be made. However, all too often, what is presented is a disguised rationale for the planners' decision.

Community Organization Needed

It is not an easy task for the public to exercise real control in areas of technical complexity and professional mystification. Individual citizen participants face a long and often lonely uphill effort. What is needed is a well developed community organization lending support and demanding that professionals play their proper role as advisors. It will take a great effort over a number of years in hundreds of communities to develop such a constituency. But the potential is there. A recent poll showed that 98 percent of the public chose good health as one of their three most important concerns; and the public is learning the true high cost of the health care they are receiving. Developing a nationwide network of health activist organizations is the challenge consumers must meet to exercise control of decisions which are, literally, a matter of life and death.

Chapter 17

THE CASE FOR PUBLIC OWNERSHIP OF MEDICAL TECHNOLOGY

John L. S. Holloman

In her autobiography, one of the earlier New York City Health Commissioners, Dr. Josephine Baker,[1] said:

> I remember how I felt when, after we had our baby health stations established and doing well in the Brownsville section of Brooklyn, a petition was forwarded to my desk from the Mayor's office signed by 30-odd Brooklyn doctors protesting bitterly against the Bureau of Child Hygiene because it was ruining medical practice by its results in keeping babies well and demanding that it be abolished in the interests of the medical profession.

Dr. Baker's response to this criticism was: "This is the first genuine compliment I have received since the Bureau was established." I have used this brief excerpt from Dr. Baker's autobiography to illustrate one aspect of the conflict between the private sector's interests and the public's right to health services.

Now, perhaps more than in Dr. Baker's time, we are seeing how difficult it is to provide for the public when private, vested interests are determining the shape of the health care delivery system.

Why Public Ownership?

A case for the public ownership of medical technologic resources is strong morally and is also eminently practical. The public already purchased the technology and gave it away to the private sector. Almost the whole of the highly technologic medical care system has been nourished, developed, and supported by public resources and public money: 88 percent of the general hospitals in the United States are either government operated or tax-exempt, private, "nonprofit voluntary" institutions. These hospitals are either supported directly by tax-levied funds or drawn from tax base by virtue of their tax-exempt status. Mainly through Medicare and Medicaid, the government now pays for more than 50 percent of the operating costs of voluntary hospitals. Thus, the public underwrites the purchase and maintenance costs of a tremendous amount of acute care technology, as well as the salaries of the interns and residents working in the hospitals. The public has also made a major commitment to the education of physicians and other health professions with more than 70 percent of the cost of professional education a gift from the taxpayer.

Many hospitals for the voluntary sector have been built by the public. Since 1946, through the Hill-Burton Act, billions of dollars have been made available by Congress for hospital construction in the private nonprofit sector. In return for these public grants, hospitals were required to provide a certain small proportion of free care to the indigent. A hospital building boom (and a great deal of what may have been unneeded construction) was stimulated by the Hill-Burton program. Very few institutions, however, lived up to their free care obligations until legal action on behalf of consumers in the 1970s forced greater hospital compliance with the law.

Much of the technology now used routinely and profitably in the practice of medicine was developed directly as a result of government sponsored research and/or tax-exempt contributions from the public.

New drug development and testing is an example. Under the supervision of the federal Food and Drug Administration, drug research on human subjects takes place throughout the country in tax-exempt and government institutions. Patent rights, designed to insure profits to the developers, are then consigned by another agency of government to those in control of the production of those pharmaceuticals. Marketing of the drug product becomes a profit-making venture for all who handle the drug's production and distribution. While the patent rights exist, the generic formula may not be manufactured, distributed or sold without purchasing written permission from the patent holders. What is the public's reward for supporting the development of this new drug treatment technology? According to a U.S. Senate committee[2] investigating the costs of drugs, the mark-up on some drugs exceeds 1400 percent. This is but one example of the public's lending a feeding hand for the development of medical technology and then getting its hand bitten in return.

Moral Right to Health Care

As a society we have said that we believe that no citizen should be barred from receiving health care services. Further, we have said that we believe that the fact of poverty should not disqualify a person from receiving high quality health care. In short, we have proclaimed health care to be a right rather than a privilege. Congress has enacted major legislation which provides health insurance for certain categories of persons. There is Medicare for older citizens and Medicaid for the poor. Through these pieces of legislation, we agreed to finance part of the health care bill for certain people. However, these partial financing arrangements have not made reality out of the rhetoric of health care rights. Health services still are not available to all citizens. In actuality, obtaining adequate health care services is still very much a privilege, and obtaining high quality and comprehensive services is still very often a matter of luck.

Estimates of the proportion of the population who are "medically indigent," not covered by Medicare or Medicaid and unable to afford private insurance, has been put as high as 30 percent. In addition, DHEW[3] reports that about 12 percent of the population has no regular source of primary care, such as a doctor or clinic. Although government has taken on some social responsibility for its citizens, the delivery of health care has been left in private hands. When vested interests continue to vigorously (and successfully) resist any structural changes in the system, it becomes impossible to fill service gaps, to guarantee quality, or to control costs. Organizational chaos, competition among providers, and the drive for profits and individual gain remain deterrents to efficiency, equity, and quality in health care. Not only have financing programs not had any significant impact on these characteristic weaknesses in the system, they have tended in some cases to reinforce some of the system's worst features. If we take seriously the idea that health care is a right, we must find a way to deliver high quality services, equally available to all people in an efficient manner.

Economic Chaos

There is the question of disorganization within our essentially private system and its impact on health and on the national budget. An indefinite delay in promised programs for national health coverage has resulted from the present economic chaos in which we find ourselves. Recent governmental administrations have engaged in several desperate and sometimes massive attempts to control rising costs in the health sector. Yet, each solution stops short of actually organizing the delivery system. Talk of putting a 9 percent "cap" on annual increases in hospital charges resulted in a predictably ineffective voluntary cost control program in the private sector. The National Health Planning and Resources Development Act of 1974, resulting in the creation of an enormous network of regional health planning agencies, was another attempt to deal with economic problems and deficiencies in health services. Again, underlying problems were left untouched.

Root causes of the expense and inequities in medical care include the crazy quilt of public and private health institutions, the variety of commercial and nonprofit insurance policies, and the myriad public programs offering partial and overlapping coverage for certain health services. As a result, we have an ungainly aggregation of health facilities and practitioners which make up our health care "system." Individual health institutions are compelled to compete with one another in order to attract attending physicians and paying patients. In this contest for survival, a tremendous amount of attractive technology is purchased and operated. Extra and inappropriate services are performed while other kinds of basic health services go unprovided.

This kind of wastefulness and duplication is a direct result of the public's open-ended financing of health care services through an unregulated and unorganized private sector. Unfortunately, the health marketplace does not seem to operate under benign economic laws which function to give the public the needed services at the best possible price. On the contrary, any and every increase in hospital operating costs and physicians' fees are guaranteed by public and private third-party insurance plans. If medical care charges go up, so do taxes and insurance premiums.

Effect on Quality of Care

As for the effect of the health care system's disorganization on quality, it is a truism to describe the care received in the system as "fragmented" and "episodic." It is also well known that needed primary and preventive services are absent. As a consequence, the overall health status of our population does not compare favorably with other developed nations of the world.

In terms of technology specifically, there have been many adverse effects on health associated with lack of coordination in the system. Utilization of existing medical technology is thought to cause an increase in the number of unnecessary procedures and in iatrogenic (physician caused) and technogenic (technology caused) illnesses. On the other hand, this same disorganization and lack of coordination in the institutional system means that some groups enjoy the advantages of advanced medical technologies while others do not. Scarce technologic resources might be more equitably distributed.

A National Health Service

Why should the government be involved in overseeing and providing health services? Government is the only credible organizational framework within which the present chaotic and fragmented systems can be unified. In a public system, profit is eliminated as an incentive and the basic motive for the system becomes the meeting of public health goals. A regionalized, public system is needed if we seriously expect to deliver comprehensive high quality health services.

In a national health service scheme, all institutions and health resources would be owned publicly. Each area would have a coordinated system of workable units in which health professionals would provide the full range of health services. In such a system, the facilities provided to each region would include: a number of health centers for primary and preventive mental and physical health services; general hospitals for acute care, a university medical center serving as the site for specialty care and tertiary level hospitalization; long-term hospitals and home care services.

Advantages of this kind of system are many. First, the public's resources can be effectively and evenly distributed among all groups in the population. Second, people can enter the system at the appropriate level of care (whether primary, acute, specialty, or long-term) and be assured of continuous, coordinated treatment. Third, since one complete set of services would be planned for each region, superfluous costs associated with competition and unnecessary duplication would be minimized. Fourth, a regionalized, public system obviates the need to administer a number of separately funded, narrowly focused programs covering certain categories of consumers (the elderly, the poor, mothers, and infants, etc.)

Purchase and distribution of medical technology through a single public system would mean that all people would have access to whatever medical technology is part of the health care arsenal of the day. Public need would be the determinant of what public money would buy. Competition among hospitals would no longer drain the public's resources.

A unitary system would also assure a more reasonable distribution of technology both among the facilities within a given service area and from region to region across the country.

As the medical arts have evolved into the medical sciences, the provision of health care has become an increasingly technologic matter. Hospital plants, the CT scanners, the kidney dialysis machines, the syringes, the vaccines are all technologic entities. Consequently, questions about the effectiveness of our health system have to do largely with the quality, allocation, and costs of medical technology.

Finally, it should simply be said that the public has already paid in great part for the development of technologic medicine. The least the public can do for itself is to decide how it might best enjoy the advantages and protect itself from technologic dangers and abuses. Public ownership of medical technology should provide the means to achieve the desired ends.

References

1. Baker, S. J. *Fighting for life.* New York: Macmillan Co., 1939, p. 138.
2. U.S. Senate Committee on the Judiciary, Subcommittee on Antitrust and Monopoly. *Study of administered prices in the drug industry.* Report No. 488 Washington, D.C.: U.S. Govt. Printing Office, June 27, 1961, pp. 46–65.
3. USDHEW, Health Resources Administration. *Health, United States 1976–1977.* DHEW Pub. No. (HRA) 77–1232, 1977. page 212.

Chapter 18

WORKSHOP SUMMARIES

WORKSHOP 1: MAKING THE WORKPLACE SAFE FOR WORKERS AND THE COMMUNITY

Panelists: Michael McCann, Ph.D.
President, Center for Occupational Hazards
New York, N.Y.

Deborah Nagin, M.P.H.
Occupational Health Program Planner, NYC Health Systems Agency

William H. White
Assistant Director (Brooklyn), NYC Health Systems Agency

Henry Velez, M.D.
Environmental Sciences Laboratory
Mt. Sinai Hospital
New York, N.Y.

A discussion of occupational health as a major health and political issue for an industrial society opened this workshop. HEW's own regulatory and monitoring agencies report 20 percent of cancers linked to occupational hazards. Other reports suggest 390,000 new cases of occupational disease a year. There is little doubt that numerous workers are affected. Deleterious effects on individual health may not be apparent for some time, but the effect on the community as with PBB in Michigan can be immediate.

Occupational illness is growing. Several factors inhibit the control of its growth. The government's research and regulatory agencies—National Institute of Occupational Safety and Health (NIOSH) and Occupational Safety and Health Administration (OSHA)—are understaffed; the regulation process itself is slow to respond and rectify abuse. The inflationary impact of controls on industry means that the business community will not voluntarily respond to statutory requirements. A lack of trained monitoring personnel and small numbers of workers at individual workplaces lessen the chance for effective hazard detection by the workers themselves.

Next, the workshop was concerned with the relationship between the health care system and occupational illness. Although occupational illness is by no means a "new" issue, it remains outside the mainstream of health care concerns. Proper screening and surveillance require organized and standardized record keeping. Doctors have little training in recognizing occupational illness and rarely take an occupational history of patients. Detection and treatment for occupational illness can require expensive, special equipment. Finally, the injured worker may not have health coverage adequate to cover the expenses of intensive screening or treatment.

Another consideration for the worker is disclosure of a work-related illness to the company doctor. An injured worker could be transferred to a lower paying position, away from a hazard rather than the company eliminating that hazard.

Worker involvement in the monitoring and control of the workplace to assure that toxic substances are eliminated is one positive strategy. However, knowledge of hazards is limited; there is no right-to-know legislation for (chemical) labeling standards and other toxic hazards.

What is the role of the HSA in enforcing and monitoring environmental and occupational issues? A panelist suggested that HSAs could initiate health goals through the project review process by establishing occupational criteria for health care institutions. Presently, project review criteria do not include concerns of health care workers. Economic and political factors involved require labor-management participation which is often difficult to achieve.

HSA could include institutional compliance with environmental and occupational safety and health standards in the project review process.

Workshop 2: Our Aging Population: Does Medical Technology Hold Any Hope?

Moderator: Nelly Peissachowitz
National Citizens Committee on Nursing Home Reform
New York, N.Y.

Panelists: Clyde Behney, M.B.A.
Senior Analyst, Health Programs
Office of Technology Assessment, U.S. Congress
Washington, D.C.

Ron Brooke
Health Care Consultant
Brookdale Center on Aging, Hunter College
New York, N.Y.

William Wolarsky, M.D.
Medical Director
Daughters of Jacob Geriatric Center
Bronx, N.Y.

Nelly Peissachowitz opened the workshop by describing the situation of the aged in the United States as indicated by national economic and social characteristics. Although the elderly represent only 10 percent of the total population, they are 25 percent of the impoverised. As people age, they *become* poor. The fragmentation of health services and the absence of preventive provisions within Medicare programs only heighten the sense of alienation and loss felt by the elderly person. Medicare and Medicaid have in some ways actually promoted the further deterioration of health services for the elderly: deductibles and "mills" contribute to the inaccessibility of decent services. Five percent of the aged in nursing homes have no opportunity to choose or affect the quality of the conditions where they are placed. Often, they are at the mercy of social service professionals who must find suitable bed space, at times far from the elderly person's community. One solution, said Ms. Peissachowitz, is to stress human concerns in medical and nursing education.

Dr. Wolarsky continued with the theme of medical education. There is no need to create yet another subspeciality of geriatrics. Internists, who usually treat the elderly, must begin the actual study of the aging process. Patient care, rather than medical care, is needed. Dr. Wolarsky outlined possible alternatives to institutionalization: the Lombardi bill in New York to provide "nursing care without walls" paid for by the state; home health care; meals on wheels; day hospitals for the rehabilitation of stroke and fracture victims; and clinics functioning within day-care centers, with the emphasis on preventive screening. The last option, he felt, is unlikely to come about.

Ron Brooke gave a brief history of medical specialization

and technology, suggesting that the "organ-oriented" pattern of medicine has not changed in 4,000 years. Medical care, he emphasized, has never been shown to affect life expectancy. However, public health measures have had a more profound affect. Our priorities are inappropriate. We spend more on medical care than we do on benefits that would improve living standards. Mr. Brooke mentioned two important ways to improve health services to the elderly: encourage the exercise of enabling legislation (Subchapter C of the State Hospital Code) for hospitals to provide day-care services for rehabilitation, socialization, and nutrition; and place nursing homes into service areas where HSAs and the community will become a "community of interest" to monitor care and advocate for patients.

Focusing on federal activities on behalf of the elderly, Mr. Behney remarked that most research funds are channeled into traditional areas such as medicine rather than human services. For instance, the National Institute of Mental Health admits that disorders associated with the aging process are ignored. A plethora of federal agencies contributes to the fragmentation of both services and benefits available to the elderly. Because the elderly are not a political force, their demands are not heard. Also, the Congressional Committee on Aging has no legislative power.

Workshop 3: Third-Party Payers: How Do (Should) They Impact on the Future of Medical Technology?

Moderator: Ben Riskin
Administrator (retired); ERM Health Center
New York, N.Y.

Panelists: Eugene Sibery,
Vice President

Blue Cross/Blue Shield of Greater New York;
New York, N.Y.

Bruce Mansdorf, M.P.A.
Deputy Director
New York State Health Planning and Development Agency
Albany, N.Y.

Donald Rubin,
President
Consumer Commission on the Accreditation of Health Services, Inc.
New York, N.Y.

Moderator Riskin questioned the need for third-party payers. He was of the opinion that the geographic redistribution of medical personnel and guaranteed health services for every citizen are the more critical issues.

Mr. Sibery traced the technologic revolution of the last 78 years, concluding that federal, corporate, and private funds continue to finance research that will bring additional wonders. Health care goals and needs cannot keep up with advances in diagnosis and treatment. New procedures, sometimes expensive and needlessly applied, combined with the proliferation of specialized manpower have contributed to uncontrollable costs. The "Blues" of Greater New York believe that availability and allocation of resources are controlling factors governing the use and total cost of health services. In 1970, they adopted a planning and reimbursement policy to eliminate surplus beds, the duplication of services, and to strengthen ambulatory care services. At the same time, they applied prospective reimbursement methods in concert with the hospital cost control law. Consumers must play their part, too. Improved health education could also help to curtail unnecessary utilization.

Mr. Mansdorf addressed the role of government in efficacy testing, the Certificate-of-Need (CON) process, the appropriate use and affordability of equipment. The CON program should be controlling the acquisition of new technologies but "loop-holes," such as private acquisition by physicians, make regional assessment difficult. Third-party reimbursement mechanisms actually stimulated the expansion of services and technology without regard to cost effectiveness. An alternative to cost control through reimbursement would be to establish an annual statewide capital expenditure limit; a finite limit on available funds would balance the acquisition of new technology with other demands on health resources. Such a proposal is before New York State lawmakers this year.

Third-party payments operate on the blank check theory according to Don Rubin. Insured consumers are unaware of service charges. Hospitals take the insurers blank check and add up the units of service. A fee-for-service system mitigates against cost containments; unwarranted and useless services are subsidized. In short, third-party payers contribute directly to inefficiency and waste. A total utilization review program by the third-party payer is in order. This program should include adequate record keeping, a profile of tissue committee results and mortality figures related to specific treatments, mandatory second opinions, a refusal to pay providers for unnecessary work, and a "hold harmless" clause so that families of patients are not sued if the provider delivers treatment that is rejected by the carrier. Third-party payers should be "watchdogs" over the quality of services as well as the use of them.

Panel-audience discussion following the presentations touched on whether or not hospitals served community needs and the extent of the impact of third-party payers on standards of service.

WORKSHOP 4: REGIONALIZATION: CONCEPTS, MYTHS, AND REALITY

Moderator: Gail Gordon, M.P.H.
Committee for a National Health Service
New York, N.Y.

Panelists: Allan Goldstein, M.D.
New York City Health Systems Agency
New York, N.Y.

Frank Grad, LL.B.
Professor of Law
Columbia University Law School
New York, N.Y.

Marvin Lieberman, Ph.D.
Executive Secretary, Committee on Medicine and Society
New York Academy of Medicine
New York, N.Y.

Moderator Gail Gordon defined regionalization as shared services or group purchasing. Her challenge to the panel: Can regionalization be implemented in our present system or is total reform necessary?

Professor Grad addressed the relationship between the CON process, as the key to planning strategy, and regionalization. The reactive nature of the CON process and the unclear definition of "need" make the goal of redistribution of services problematic. Professor Grad emphasized that the planning law encompasses areawide planning but neglects local, autonomous control. CON, as the "cutting edge" of planning, is blunted by the mix of local, regional, and federal definitions of regionalization.

Dr. Goldstein basically concurred with the view that the lack of standard designations, such as definitions of primary, secondary, and tertiary levels of care, demands that planners work from hard data to confront each issue on its own merits. He presented three possible planning strategies for regionalization: the geographic division of services, a division of service categories, or the designation of the three levels of care. While the standardization of regional terms, for example, may help planners decide "what" to do, it will not necessarily tell them "how" to do it.

"Is regionalization possible under our system?" asked Dr. Lieberman. He cited the British approach to regionalization and concluded that it could not be applied within our present economic structure. He cautioned against tripping over definitions of regionalization. The ultimate goal of improved access may not be reached through regionalization. He noted that the price of regionalization to the British was domination by a medical elite. Our approach to health planning, he said, both reflects and promotes the pluralism of our society. He balanced the British regionalized system with its elite domination against a less than ideal regionalization responsive to consumers.

Several provocative questions came for the audience following the panel presentations. In answer to a query about consumer power within an HSA and regionalization, Dr. Grad responded that at the local level consumers may confront provider interests, at the national level consumers must face each other. Again, a question surfaced about regionalization and a national health service. Dr. Goldstein replied that HSA was committed to the idea of regionalization without a national health service. Professor Grad agreed that regionalization must proceed although a national health insurance will appear eventually.

A question about the dominance of the HSA staff and providers in decision making brought two responses. Dr. Goldstein said he was weary of complaints about staff-provider dominance. HSA records show geographic solidarity rather than consumer-provider splits. Dr. Lieberman thought a weakness was inadequate consumer leadership; perhaps paid consumer advocates would be one solution.

NAME INDEX

SUBJECT INDEX